Losing Weight in Six Days

Losing Weight in Six Days

A Case of the White Horse Island Life Detective Service

A Novel

JAY KIMIECIK AND DOUG NEWBURG

This is a work of fiction. Names, characters, places, and incidents either are the product of the authors' imaginations or are used fictitiously. Any resemblance to actual persons, living or dead, events, or locales is entirely coincidental.

Book Cover and Illustrations by Greg LaFever

ISBN-13: 9781523730834
ISBN-10: 1523730838

*Once upon a time, there was a woman who
discovered she had turned into the wrong person.*

—ANNE TYLER,
Back When We Were Grownups

*Ten thousand white horses
Will rise from the sea.
I wonder where
They'll carry me.*

*I'll try to catch a few thousand
And ride them to shore,
Ten thousand white horses
And more.*

*From out of the white caps,
The horses now come.
They're skirting, flirting,
Proceeding, receding.*

*The little ones whisper,
"Come play!"
As they quickly
Are slipping away.*

—BETSY B. LEE,
10,000 White Horses

Table of Contents

Day 4 Know

Day 5 Trust

Day 6 Create

Losing Weight in Six Days

ARRIVAL

The woman's name was Annie and when she tried to lose weight, she gained more.

Annie was like a lot of women her age: a working professional, mom to two teenagers one of whom had just started college, and wife to a man she loved at one time but now...not so sure. She hadn't had sex in months. She didn't feel like the same person anymore and the weight of it all was weighing her down. She knew something was happening to her body, her mind, her spirit. Her body felt heavy, her mind distracted, and her spirit empty. Few people picked up on how she was *really* feeling, including Annie herself.

And yet there was something about Annie that had attracted Billy to her case, something that he had recognized years ago. He knew the promise was still there, buried deep inside.

As Annie drove over the bridge that was the entry to White Horse Island, she felt different. She pulled out the scrunchy and shook her hair. She was looking forward to a fun week at the beach with her two best friends and minimal life distractions. And she was hopeful that the Spa and some time away could finally get her on the path to losing weight.

*A*nnie arrived at the White Horse Island rental house and immediately was captivated by the mellifluous sound of the ocean waves. With nightfall approaching, she was glad she had made the four and one half hours drive, even fighting Friday traffic, so that she could catch the sunrise in the morning—before her friends arrived later in the day to begin their reunion vacation week. The key was supposed to be under the ornamental turtle—it wasn't. "Damn," she muttered.

Of course, Annie checked again as if the first look might have been a mistake. No key. She hadn't planned for this. Her Outer Banks YMCA friend knew a friend who owned the house and had agreed to rent it at a steep discount to Annie and her two friends for the week as mid September was post-peak season. She tried her friend's cell but no answer.

Befuddled, Annie looked around to catch her bearings. As she turned to the sound side, she spotted in the distance what she assumed was the *White Horse Island Resort & Spa*, and then her eyes narrowed as she saw what could only be called a shack much closer to home—right next door.

What in the world, she wondered, how can that thing still be standing amongst all these beautiful homes?

Two men were sitting on the front stoop and they seemed to be watching her for their own amusement. They caught her looking and waved. She didn't want to encourage them and didn't wave back.

She was hoping they might go inside but minutes later after she had checked around the house for other possible entries—without any luck—she looked over again. This time they were waving for her to come over.

O Lord, she thought. Woman vacationer murdered on White Horse Island. Well, I don't have any other options, as she walked slowly toward the shack.

"Hi, my name's Annie. Do you guys live here?" She had decided that being forthright and aggressive was her best move.

"You might say that," the bigger of the two men answered.

"And we know your name is Annie," the little man said.

"How do you know that?"

"Bob told us you were coming," the little man said.

"He did? Why? You know, Bob?"

"Bob is one of my former clients," the big guy said. "He thought you might enjoy meeting us. We've been hanging out waiting for your arrival."

"Do you want a beer?" the little guy asked. He was wearing dark wrap-around shades, which seemed a little odd to Annie since the sun had already set. Both of them seemed to be around her age. Kinda cute, she thought, especially the big one.

"Uh...no...thanks. There was supposed to be a key left for me but it's not where Bob said it would be."

"I think Doc has it," the big guy said.

"Who's Doc?"

"I am," the little guy said. "Bob decided to give it to me for safe keeping." Doc dug in his jeans pocket, pulled out the key, and held it up like it was a rabbit pulled out of a hat.

As Annie moved closer, Doc stood up and put the key in her hand. He shook her other hand: "Hi, I'm Doc, welcome to White Horse Island."

"Hello, Doc." Annie felt a little flushed. "Who's your friend here?" pointing to the big guy.

"That's, Billy. Billy Hamilton. He's an asshole." Billy disregarded the disparaging comment and stood up to shake Annie's hand. She was surprised by the size and strength of his hand. His chest was enormous. Annie felt a tingling sensation when her hand touched his.

Breaking the awkward silence, Annie asked again, "So do you both live here?"

"Billy lives here more or less," Doc replied. "I'm just visiting for the week to help Billy with a case."

"A case, what kind of case?" asked Annie. "What are you guys private detectives or something?"

"Something like that," Doc said.

"I work on *very* private cases," Billy added.

It seemed to Annie that the guys didn't want to divulge specifics of whatever kind of case they were working on so she didn't push even though she was curious. What kind of case could they possibly be working on at a vacation spot? she wondered. "Well, it's been nice meeting you both. I'm sure I'll be seeing you during the week."

"I'm sure you will," Doc said.

Annie turned and headed back to the big house.

Billy turned to Doc: "What do you think? Think she knows what's going on?"

"I don't think so," said Doc, sounding uncertain. "We have our work cut out for us. She didn't even comment on your lame sign or the swing. I don't think she even saw them."

"You worry too much. She's just not paying attention yet. That's your job, to make her pay attention," Billy said as he turned to walk back inside the ramshackle quarters that served as the home of the newly created *White Horse Island Life Detective Service.* "Just remember you're helping with this case because you know this stuff."

"That's comforting. You are going to be around to help, right Billy?" Doc asked, but Billy had already closed the door, leaving Doc alone to ponder the challenge that lay before him. "Six days, yeah right," Doc mumbled to himself. "You're good Billy Hamilton but I wonder if you're that good."

On her way back to the house, Annie's cell rang. She recognized the number.

"Hi, Bob."

"Hey, Annie. I see you called. Did you find the key under the turtle?"

"No, Doc and Billy had it. They said you gave it to them."

"Who?"

"Doc and Billy, you know, the guys living in that shack next door."

"I don't know any Doc or Billy," Bob said. "What the hell were they doing with the house key?"

"Calm down, Bob. You don't know them?"

"No. Geez, Annie, be careful."

"Well, they seemed pretty harmless. Kinda cute actually, especially the big guy."

"Do you want me to call the police or anything?"

"No, I'll be fine. Just let me get settled in. I'll call ya later."

Annie tried the key and to her relief it worked. The whole key thing had her a little shook up but there was something about Doc and Billy that kept her from panicking. They seemed harmless but she made a mental note to ask why they had lied about the house key. After bringing in her suitcase and the doggie bag container from the restaurant in town, she did lock the front door, checked all the other doors to make sure they were locked, and gave Bob a quick call to ease his mind.

After she hung up, Annie wondered how Doc and Billy knew her name if they didn't know Bob.

The rental house was exquisite. How do people afford these monstrosities, Annie wondered, as she turned on every light and explored every room? She chose the bedroom on the third floor overlooking the ocean. Early bird catches the worm, she thought.

Opening the window, she breathed in the ocean air deep into her lungs. She stood there for a long time enjoying the moment as the moon pierced the beach darkness with light. Now this feels good. She opened the double doors that led her out to a beautiful, three-tiered deck with stairs leading down to the beach. The waves had a rhythm to them. She leaned on the rail and just listened. I don't have this, she thought. My life has no rhythm. Every day seems like some new crisis to deal with. Her teen son was driving her crazy: anxiety attacks, smoking pot, bad grades. The work at the Y was getting stressful and who knows what Maggie was doing in college. Annie hoped her daughter wasn't doing what she did in college.

Her thoughts were interrupted by what sounded like thunder coming from the beach below. At first it looked like moving shadows on the sand. But after a second or two she realized the shadows were actually horses galloping. Annie gasped and watched in amazement as the small herd thundered by. The lead horse was white. And then they were gone with only the sound of their pounding hooves in their wake. Annie was stunned by the power and beauty of what she had just seen and felt a sense of freedom and power pulse through her body. After waiting a few minutes for a possible return by the horses, which didn't happen, she went back inside to unpack. She prepared for bed but even the Patricia Cornwell novel couldn't keep her thoughts from wondering about the horses. So powerful, so free. Finally, she lulled herself to sleep with thoughts about getting up early enough to catch the sunrise.

Day 1
Touch

One

The Game With No Name

Annie saw the White Horses rise out of the waves and thunder toward her on the beach, but she wasn't afraid. As they approached her, they started whinnying, which turned into chants of her name: "Annie… Annie…Annie…" She joined in with the chants and then jumped up on one of the horses and rode back into the ocean….

Annie's dreamlike state was shattered by human laughter and grunts and voices. She lay in bed, her mind working hard to determine what was dream and what was reality. As she began to rouse, she realized where she was and that the sounds were coming from the beach. Feeling a bit perturbed that her deep sleep had been interrupted, she pulled on a pair of shorts and a polo shirt and walked out on the deck. The brilliant sunlight that greeted her saddened her a bit as she realized she missed its daily birth.

Shading her eyes from the sun, she zoomed in on the noisemakers. About 10 people were doing something on the beach that she couldn't figure out right away. They seemed to be playing some kind of game. One guy had a beach ball held between his legs and was hopping wildly toward a couple of cones 10 to 20 yards away. As he neared the goal, a big guy came up and blindsided him, leading with his chest. The guy with the ball went flying and splattered face first into the sand. The hit was so vicious that Annie flinched. The big guy placed the loose ball between his legs and headed in the other direction with other players hopping after him. The guy who got hammered sat up, shook his head, brushed the sand from his hair and face, and smiled. When he picked up his sunglasses, Annie realized it was Doc. The big guy with the ball was Billy. No one could catch him and as he reached the other goal he raised his hands over his head, signaling touchdown. Billy had a big grin and his teammates pounded him in jubilation. It looked like Billy's team had just won.

Where did these people come from? Annie wondered. They all looked pretty fit, even the couple of women playing, who looked to be about her age, seemed in good shape. She envied them. Where do they get the energy?

Billy spotted Annie watching and waved. Annie, embarrassed, gave a mini-wave back. "C'MON DOWN AND PLAY," Billy shouted. Annie shook her head and yelled back: "MAYBE LATER." As Billy shook his hand at her in mock disgust, Doc nailed him with a headlong run that ended with Doc falling backwards into the sand. Billy threw the ball at him and kept walking. From his flat-on-his-back position, Doc raised his arms and then his two middle fingers, which made Annie smile.

Who are these guys, she wondered, and then went back inside to start her day.

*B*eing alone was not something that Annie did much anymore. She didn't particularly like being by herself so she filled up her day. She was always in meetings with her Y staff or the board or raising money. At home, she was barely coping with her teenage son or with her husband, who seemed most interested in doing things that didn't involve her: golf, running, and watching every sporting event possible on TV. She missed her daughter.

She foraged through the kitchen getting her bearings, found some Green Mountain Coffee, and got the coffee maker going. The view from the kitchen was spectacular and she could see that Billy and the boys were playing another game, this one involving the water. The first sip made her remember that she had the leftover pancakes in the frig from her stop at *Stack 'em High* in the town of White Horse yesterday evening before arriving at the rental home. After heating them up and finishing them off (without syrup), she ventured upstairs for her shower to get ready for her pampering at the Spa that her two friends had purchased for her as her reward for finding and booking the rental house.

Two of Annie's best friends from high school and college had talked her into a trip to the Outer Banks to celebrate their 30th high school reunion. At first, Annie wasn't too keen on the idea but after talking with Bob who said he had access to the "perfect house," she decided to venture out of Charlottesville for her first adventure to the Outer Banks. Sam and Kate would be arriving later today to begin a week of reminiscing, margaritas, and lying on the beach.

The shower felt good and as she stepped out she caught a quick reflection of herself in the full-length mirror on the back of the bathroom door. "God, I'm fat," she declared matter of fact, immediately covering herself back up with the towel. Her weight was the one aspect of her life she felt no control over. She had tried and tried and tried...and failed. Annie had gained the weight during her pregnancies and could never get back to her pre-pregnancy weight. Thirty years removed from high school she was now almost exactly 30 pounds over her high school tennis playing weight. She had tried the diets, the low-fat foods, combo drugs, cutting down the portion sizes, you name it. After awhile, it had become easier and easier to buy replacement clothes to hide her growing frame than exercise and eat the way the experts told her she should. What made it worse was that for the past 25 years she worked at the Charlottesville YMCA, and for the last five years, was its executive director. For cripes sake, she thought, I work at the Y. I should be able to figure this out. But she hadn't, just like the thousands of people who had joined her Y over the years and then dropped out. Not to mention all of those people who were too afraid to even join. She rarely worked out in the Y's fitness room and things like tennis, golf, and running were more difficult with the extra weight to lug around.

Annie put on her one-piece swimsuit that in her own words made her look like a "beached whale." She covered up with shorts, a long-sleeve shirt, her sun hat, and tennis shoes, and ventured outside to put the key under the turtle in case the girls arrived before her return. Curious, she strolled around back to see what the beach was like. She came to a paved path and stopped to catch her bearings. It looked like the path wound all the way to the Spa, which was her next stop, and all the way to town in the other direction. The path seemed never ending in both directions. She caught a glimpse of Billy's shack. It looked even worse in the daylight—balls and boogie boards were strewn all over as if a bunch of little kids had been let loose to play and not forced to clean up. Looking to the ocean, the game gang was now playing in the water but it looked like Billy was just sitting in his chair. The game started to annoy her a bit and the incident with the key was beginning to get under her craw. She had plenty of time before her Spa appointment. Time for some answers. Annie stepped off the path and headed for Billy.

She didn't know it then but Billy and Doc wanted Annie to step off the path. She had to step off the path. It was the only way to lose weight. And she had only six days to do it.

Billy was simply watching the others, relaxing. He was sweaty, sitting in the water, his right leg straight out resting on top of his left leg, his arms behind him, his hands buried in the sand, arms close to hyperextension.

Billy couldn't hear Annie's "hello" from behind him so she re-positioned herself at the tip of his toes and said a louder "HELLO." No response. "EXCUSE ME, BUT WHAT ARE YOU GUYS DOING?"

"Playing," Billy said without looking up at her. He tilted his head toward a bunch of lines and numbers drawn in the sand higher up on the beach, just below the high tide line.

Annie looked at the numbers and lines.

"Playing what?" she asked softly, feeling a bit embarrassed.

"*The Game With No Name*. Wanna play?" he said, still not looking at her. Then he leaned forward and looked at Annie through one open eye. He smiled a cocky smile.

"What? Annie asked, confused. "Uh…no…I have an appointment at the Spa in a bit."

"Ooh. Aren't we special? Massage?"

"Well, no. A wellness coach first, then some pampering."

"So what are you playing that you need a coach?" Billy asked as he looked past her out to the water to see how the game was going.

"What?" Annie asked again. Billy had caught her off guard. This conversation was not going how Annie had envisioned. She was mired in confusing thoughts.

Billy took the silence as his opportunity to join the game. "Gotta go." Billy smiled as he jumped up and ran into the water.

Frustrated, Annie watched the game for a few minutes and deep down wished she was playing the game instead of going to the Spa. The spot had been touched, if only for a brief moment. She headed back to the path that would take her to the Spa.

*D*oc, sitting on the weathered deck in the back of the Shack, had witnessed the exchange between Annie and Billy. As he watched Annie walk back to the path, he knew exactly how she felt. Billy Hamilton was the most exasperating person he had ever met, but he was also the most relentless. Billy talked in what was like another language and lived a life that seemed foreign to most. He lived true to how he felt and Billy was the most authentic person Doc knew. They had tried to work together over the years to share what Billy knew and lived without much success. Ironically, Doc believed the stress of it all got him sick. Billy was always on to the next permutation of the process while Doc was still trying to figure out how to interpret the "old" stuff. It was a recipe for professional disaster. He hoped this time it would be different. It had to be. He could not fail and let himself or Billy down.

"Hi Annie," Doc said softly to muffle the sound.

Hearing the voice and her name startled Annie who had had her head down and was walking with a purpose on the path to the Spa. She did a 360 trying to pinpoint the sound and in the process her sunglasses fell on the path.

She heard "Where you headed?" as she bent over to pick them up and was finally able to turn toward the sound.

"Oh, Doc, you startled me," she said, as she recognized his huge wrap-around shades.

"I didn't mean to." Lying. He needed her attention. "What's up?"

"Oh, I'm just going to the Spa."

"Cool. That should be fun."

Annie nodded.

Doc waited. Billy always told him not to be afraid of the silence. If anything, Doc was a good student.

Annie was getting a good vibe from this funny little man with the big shades. She also had some questions.

"Do you want to sit down for a bit?" Doc asked, positioning the chair next to him to make conversation easier.

"Well…uh…okay. I have some time before my appointment."

"I see you were talking with Billy," Doc said as Annie sat down.

"Oh…yea. He's a real character," Annie replied as she noticed a big bruise on Doc's arm. She couldn't help herself: "Is that where Billy hit you this morning?" pointing to the bruise.

"Yea, yea, just part of the game. It's nothing."

"What kind of game was that? Annie asked.

"*The Game With No Name,*" Doc responded.

"That's the game Billy said they are playing now. What does that mean?"

"It's pretty simple, really," said Doc, leaning forward. "The game we were playing earlier we call Sandstorm. I think the game they're playing now is Nitro Waterball. The name of the game isn't all that important but we have fun naming each one we come up with."

"Well, I've never heard of those games."

"I know. We make them up. They don't exist until we create them thereby *The Game With No Name*."

"But what's the point?"

"Do they look like fun?" asked Doc.

"Well, yea, but that Sandstorm game seemed a little dangerous. I mean you got pummeled by Billy."

"Just part of playing the game. When *you* create the game you kinda know what you're getting yourself into."

"Interesting."

Silence, except for the waves. Annie looked out toward the ocean. Wild horses, games with crazy names, two guys in a shack. Not the way she had envisioned her week at White Horse to begin. But she had a feeling that she was being drawn into something. The beach was alive with something, with what she wasn't exactly sure. But something was touching her in a way she hadn't felt in years.

Annie finally broke the silence: "So, you guys seem pretty harmless but why did you lie to me about knowing Bob and saying that he gave you the key to the rental house? I talked to him yesterday and he says he doesn't know you guys and that he certainly didn't give you the key."

"That's odd. I'm pretty sure Billy knows Bob. But we took the key mostly to get your attention."

"My attention? What do you mean?"

Doc hesitated. His life had been full of hesitation and worry. He was sick of it and probably sick from it. What the hell.

"Well...we don't have much time," Doc began. "We took the key to get your attention. You probably won't believe me but basically Billy is a... well...a life detective for lack of a better term." Doc couldn't believe he was saying this. "Billy has taken on your case and he brought me in to help."

"My case?" Annie replied in between nervous laughter. "My case? What are you talking about? I don't have a case for you guys to work on. I'm here on vacation."

"Well, not really. You're at White Horse to lose weight."

Annie was thrown off guard by Doc's statement and stopped laughing, taking a moment to collect herself. "So, you're telling me that you and Billy are life detectives and that you are on my case, literally, to help me lose weight. I don't believe this. You're looney."

"Well, Billy's the real life detective. He's the best. I'm just here to help because I believe in him and I know a thing or two about losing weight. You do want to lose weight, right?"

"Well, yes, but I wouldn't call it my case," Annie retorted.

"Well, that's what we're calling it." Doc replied, getting a little agitated.

"I think you're both deranged," Annie said as she rose to leave. "I don't know how you know me and I definitely don't need your help. It's not like I hired you guys to help me or anything. I have to get to my Spa appointment," Annie said defiantly and turned to walk away on the path to the Spa.

Doc scrambled to his feet. Think. Think. Think. Touch, Touch, Touch.

"ANNIE, JUST MAKE SURE YOU TAKE A GOOD LOOK OUT TO THE OCEAN," Doc shouted in her direction. He wasn't sure if she heard him or not. He watched helplessly as Annie walked down the path. That went well, Doc thought, as he slumped back down in the chair.

Look out to the ocean? Annie wondered. Losing weight? My case? Annie felt confused. How did Doc know she wanted to lose weight? Well, that one was pretty obvious. But how did he know her at all? And just how were these two guys in a dilapidated shack supposed to help her? Stealing a key to get caught? What the hell. Look out to the ocean?

Look out to the ocean.

Annie slowed her pace and then abruptly stopped. She turned toward the water. At first, she just saw a blending of sun, sky, and water. But as her eyes adjusted, she spotted *The Game With No Name* gang still playing in the water. This time it looked like they were using a tennis ball and timing throws to coincide with a wave crashing into the receiver just as the ball arrived. Of course, this made it more challenging—and more fun. She saw Billy, sitting in a beach chair, flip a stick backwards over his head to a yellow lab that ran to fetch it. The dog returned the stick to Billy's lap and then waited patiently for the next flip. Four young children were running along the beach with the lead girl holding string to a kite that was riding the air behind her. The other kids were jumping and running trying to touch the kite. Then Annie spotted the pelicans. A pod of them were gliding along, just above the water. Annie was mesmerized. How beautiful, she thought. She watched till they disappeared where water met sky.

Annie smiled and took a deep breath. She felt more relaxed. Then she realized she was going to be late for her Spa appointment and began a fast walk on the path.

Doc didn't take his eyes off Annie until she disappeared around a bend in the path.

*D*oc saw Billy walking toward him and braced himself mentally for the conversation.

"How did it go?" Billy asked as he eased himself into the other chair. Obi, the lab, shook himself dry at Doc's expense.

"Are you sure we have the right case, Billy?" Doc asked.

"That well, huh," Billy grunted. "And yes we have the right case."

"Well, remind me again, Sherlock, just how are we going to crack this case?" Doc asked.

"You know the answer. I don't know why I have to keep drumming it into you. It's tiring." Billy wished Doc would trust himself as much as he trusted in him. "Just keep it simple. How people feel determines how they perform. You're the one who made the connection between feel and healthy living. That's why you're here."

"You're right. I'm just not sure I've got it in me anymore." Doc removed his sunglasses and put a few drops in his eyes, which were irritated and red, from a small capsule he had removed from his shorts pocket.

"Yes, you do" is all Billy said.

"Well, I'm a little tired. I'm going inside to rest a bit," Doc said.

"Just remember, Doc, today is about touching that clean, unspoiled spot. Annie needs to reawaken it before anything else can happen."

"I know," Doc replied as he walked into the shack. But I have no foggy idea how to do that, Doc thought, as he crashed on to the couch.

During her walk to the Spa, Annie couldn't get Doc and Billy out of her thoughts. Fun images of playing on the beach flashed through her mind. She couldn't explain it but she felt different.

As spas go, this was upper-middle class. Designed to attract more money to White Horse Island, it catered to the suburban moms who'd been vacationing at the island for decades. They embraced and nurtured the idea of being "Mom." The week or two they spent at the beach was a coming together of family—barbecues, men doing man things, women doing woman things. Shopping was a sport on beaches like this throughout the world and over the last ten or fifteen years, it dominated the WHI's economy. Several women sauntered around a large square reception area. They were all wearing white robes with white slippers, carrying large white bath sheets. Everything is white, Annie thought. She felt out of place, nervous. The place was too clinical, like a doctor's office.

"Can I help you?" said the disinterested, young blonde manning the reception area.

Annie just stood there taking it in…not ready to give in to the spa experience her well-meaning friends had signed her up for. She looked at the receptionist, disdainful of her youth. She felt her lungs take a breath and gathered herself, which was when she noticed the heavy make-up the receptionist was wearing. She'd probably had a hard night of partying.

Annie wanted to know where she'd been the night before, her contempt turning to curiosity and empathy.

"Uh...no, thanks, I'm just looking around," Annie replied, deciding she wasn't ready to reveal that she had an appointment.

Annie noticed a group of rattan chairs that wrapped around a small fountain, the water seeming to come out of no where, a gentle sound as it ran off the rocks and back into a small pool built into the Mexican tile floor. Annie did not like anything about how all of this felt. She glanced back at the receptionist and determined that she wasn't really blonde. The side tables were covered with yoga and self help magazines. Annie just laughed as she looked at the titles of the articles about finding happiness and inner peace. She was laughing at herself, how stupid she felt that her life had led her to this kind of place. But here she was.

She wanted to walk out, to run away really. While contemplating this action, she heard pop...pop...pop...pop...pop...coming from somewhere outside. Walking out she followed the sound till she spotted the nearby tennis courts and a woman who looked to be about Annie's age hitting forehands off a machine. She would know that sweet sound anywhere as ball met racket. The courts were clay. Annie had always wondered what it would be like to play on a clay court. She thought about the many hours she had spent on the courts of her youth. She could almost feel herself moving, swinging, grunting. Bone tired but full of life.

With a touch of wistfulness Annie turned to head back to the Spa and her appointment. But the wonder of nature's whisper was calling her to play. She was drawn to the water, not the Spa. *The Game With No Name.* Tennis balls. Pelicans. She blew off her appointment and headed back to the house.

*B*illy saw Annie coming down the path. She was skipping, like a little girl.

"What are you all happy about?" asked Billy, as Annie approached the shack.

Again, Annie was at first confused as to where the voice was coming from?

"Do you always walk on the path?" Billy followed-up.

From the second question Annie was able to locate the voice and turned towards it. "Oh, Billy, you scared me," said Annie, recognizing the man sitting in a chair on the deck of the shack. Boy, do you ever scare me, thought Annie. But her attraction to Billy was so strong she wanted to reach out and touch him. "You and Doc have a way of interrupting people," Annie said, trying not to appear flustered.

"Yea, I've been told that. Most people need to be interrupted even thought they don't like it at first."

"Do I need to be interrupted?" asked Annie.

"Well, have you touched anything lately?" asked Billy, pulling over a chair as an invitation for Annie to sit down.

"What do you mean?" Annie asked, as she sat down across from Billy. She loved his chest, and his hands; his hands were so big, so inviting to hold.

"Has anything touched you lately in a way to give you goose bumps or make you wonder or feel vital, alive, free?"

"Well, I was just skipping. That felt good. Haven't done that in awhile."

"But you were doing it on the path."

"So?"

"That was my second question, "Do you always walk on the path?""

"I'm not sure what that means. Is there some kind of double meaning or voodoo philosophy that you're hitting me with here?"

"It's a simple question?"

"Well, it doesn't sound simple to me," Annie said. She was getting more aggravated and more attracted to Billy at the same time. "Okay, yes, I pretty much always walk on the path."

"Why?"

"I don't know. It's easy I guess."

"When you were younger, where did you skip?"

"Everywhere."

"Right, and so that way you never just touched things in your immedi-ate reach, limiting your life. You felt all of it. Walking, even skipping on the path, limits your ability to touch what's right about you, and believe me, there's a lot that's right about you."

"I'll take that as a compliment."

"More of an observation."

"Well, thanks…I think," said Annie.

"Look, we are all born with the power to touch, to touch that clean, unspoiled spot. And we do it, most of us, when we're younger. Then we get on the path and forget about it. Or we're told to stop, to act our age. You want to try something?"

"What?"

"Take your shoes off and before you get to your house, skip around anywhere but on the path and see what that feels like."

"But that's silly."

"Whatever. Just try it."

Annie looked around to see if anyone was watching.

"And what's the point of this?" Annie asked, still unsure she wanted to go barefoot.

"I think you already know," Billy replied. "Gotta go," he said as he got up to go inside.

Annie looked around one more time, took off her shoes, held them in her hands, and took off. Barefoot, she skipped in the sand, heading for the water. Sand flew everywhere. She skipped at the water line, with water splashing in every direction, before turning back towards the house. For some reason, she leaped over the path and skipped some more before stop-ping as she reached her front door.

She stopped to regroup. That was fun, she thought. I felt free, and I'm amazed I just did that. Annie's thoughts shifted back to Billy. Her attrac-tion to this big, strange man was unsettling. And she didn't know whether to laugh or cry about the strange goings on since she arrived at White Horse Island. She spotted the new car in the drive, and was glad that Sam and Kate were here to take her mind off her case—whatever in the hell that meant. She wasn't sure if she would tell them about what was going on or not, even though Annie had known them for over 30 years—dating back to elementary school and, later, their high school tennis days, and then in college. Both Kate and Sam had left Charlottesville after college and had found good careers. Both divorced, she was a little concerned about them finding Billy, especially Sam, who attracted men like kids to ice cream. Just before opening the door, Annie mustered up the best fake smile she could.

"Hello, anybody home?" Annie called out, as she dropped her shoes.

"Is that Annie Oakley," a voice cried out from the kitchen.

"Is that Lil Orphan Annie," another voice echoed.

Kate and Sam dashed into the foyer and gave Annie the good ole group hug. Annie couldn't help but flash a real smile. These were her best friends from high school and college. Though they had drifted away a bit over the years, they were still tight. They kept in touch on Facebook and were sure to hook up when travel took them to each other's home city.

Annie was the first to pull away.

"So what have you fine ladies been up to?" Annie asked.

"The trip was great. We met at the airport, picked up the rental, and drove in. We stocked up on some groceries in town, and here we are," said Sam, who looked as great as ever. "Great job on the house, Annie. It's spectacular."

"I don't know about you two, but I've been looking forward to this for months," said Kate. "Who is ready for some lunch and my world-famous margaritas?"

Both Sam and Annie raised their hands in unison.

After devouring the spread that Kate whipped up, the margaritas were going down like candy. Conversation revolved around the families, Sam's sexual escapades, and life at work. Annie felt the buzz. Felt good. Good friends with a view of the ocean. What could be better?

"So what are we going to do this week?" Kate asked.

"Nothing but the beach and margaritas," said Sam.

"Did you guys notice that shack next door? What is up with that place?" asked Kate.

"I've met the guys who are staying there. They seem pretty harmless." Annie said, trying too hard to sound disinterested.

"Well, do tell me more," said Sam.

"There's not much more to tell," said Annie. "I just met them briefly when I was walking around."

"So that reminds me. How was the Spa?" asked Kate.

"It was good. Great massage. Thanks for setting that up for me." Annie just couldn't break the news that she bolted the Spa. She was still surprised by her actions. She glanced out the window and saw that the boys were in action again. Don't they ever get tired? She was hoping that Sam and Kate wouldn't see them. She really didn't want to have to explain the whole affair. How do you explain that a couple of guys who you don't know are staying next door to help you lose weight? Ridiculous.

The drinking and reminiscing continued through late afternoon until the effects of Kate's margaritas led to each of them passing out on the sofa.

Two

PELICAN STEW

Annie woke first and immediately felt the need for a shower to help her come back to life. She headed upstairs to her room, grabbed the shoebox from her suitcase, and laid it on the bed. Annie stared at the shoebox, not quite sure why she brought it, or more importantly, why she brought what was in it. Finally, she opened the top slowly, as if she didn't know what was inside, and began riffling through the myriad pictures. She was looking for one in particular—a team tennis picture from their high school days. There it was. In the photo Annie was holding up a team trophy with her teammates, Kate and Sam, by her side. She flipped to the back: "*To my favorite tennis player. Never lose that smile, Annie,*" Coach Anderson had scribbled. Annie noticed her smile. It's so big. Where did my smile go? A tear ran down her cheek. This is crazy, she thought. I shouldn't be crying over a silly high school picture. I have a good life. But where did my smile go?

The shower made Annie's head feel almost normal. As she lost herself in the post-shower routine, it took her a few minutes to realize that the pulsating music she was hearing was coming from the beach. Venturing out to the deck, she saw Billy hovering over a fire pit. He was stirring something in a pot surrounded by other would-be chefs. Jackson Browne's *Pretender* was loud enough to be heard up and down the beach. But what really got her attention were the two guys in Crocodile Dundee-type hats aiming bows and arrows at what appeared to be replicas of wild boars stationed near the water. Am I still drunk? she wondered. Billy spotted her and waved for her to come down. "Guess not," she muttered to herself. "You're damn right I'm coming down. This has gone far enough."

———❦———

Annie hustled downstairs past the lifeless bodies of Kate and Sam and headed out back to the beach. She was pretty sure you couldn't cook in a fire pit on the beach and she was absolutely positive you couldn't shoot arrows. And obviously the music volume was way too high. Annie was at WHI to relax, to forget about life for a while. That was hardly the way it was going her first 24 hours.

Billy saw her coming. He could tell she had confrontation on her mind.

"I guess we got your attention," he said as she approached. "Do you want some Pelican Stew?"

"Pelicans? Now you're killing pelicans?" Annie cried out.

"Hey, Billy, is this Annie, the woman you were telling us about?" said one of the boar killers.

Billy put his finger to his lips as the signal to zip it.

Annie was incredulous.

"Nice to meet you, Annie. My name's Ian," said the man as he extended the tip of his bow for her to shake. "Billy said he was going to cook some Peli Stew for you. We'll let you have first dibs. We all believe it's ready but Billy always makes us wait. Drives us nuts."

Annie looked around at the other famished diners.

"But, you can't kill and eat Pelicans can you?" Annie asked.

The laughter from the group almost drowned out the blaring music.

"Pelicans?" The other bow and arrow man exclaimed. "It's chicken."

"Then why do you call it Pelican Stew? Annie asked.

"That's Billy's nickname," said Doc as he broke through the crowd. "Billy Pelican. Get it. Bill...eeh...Pelican. His nose is about as big as a pelican's bill."

Now it was Annie's turn to laugh out loud. She hadn't caught herself laughing in awhile.

"Hey, Annie, do you want to take a crack at the boars while we wait?" Ian asked.

"No offense to you guys, but you can't really cook over an open fire on the beach here and I'm sure you can't be shooting arrows at fake wild boars while blasting music." Annie exclaimed. "It doesn't seem safe."

"What do you mean?" Billy asked.

"Well, I'm sure it's against the rules."

"So. Have you never broken any rules?"

"Well, probably, but I'm sure this is illegal. I mean you could kill someone."

Now it was Billy's turn to laugh.

"Ian and Mac are national champion field archers. They could shoot an apple off your head if you let them." Billy replied. "You should try it."

"I don't want to stand with an apple on my head," said Annie.

"No, I mean try the bow and arrow." Billy said. "Stew will be ready shortly. Do you want some stew?"

Annie thought of Kate and Sam passed out in the house. "Uh…sure… I guess." She was feeling a bit better about the situation and Ian and Mac seemed as harmless as Doc and Billy.

Ian gave Annie a quick tutorial on shooting with a bow and then demonstrated with a few shots, striking the heart of the boar each time. She was amazed by his skill. They moved in closer for Annie. She tried several times—one arrow flew into the ocean, another buried in the sand. But she did strike the boar's butt on one of her attempts and Ian and Mac clapped. Annie was impressed with herself.

"Not bad, not bad," said Ian. "You've got some hidden skills."

"So how do you guys know Billy?" Annie asked as they walked to gather up the arrows.

"Well, that's a long story," said Mac, but the short of it is that about 10 years ago, Ian and me somehow found Billy. We had been hunting with bows and were looking for something that didn't involve, you know, actually killing real animals. So we started doing this field archery where you shoot at targets in the woods and some of it involved shooting at these fake creatures."

"You mean there are actually competitions for this? Annie asked.

"Oh sure, it's big, especially in Europe." Ian replied. "You shoot at all kinds of animals: lions, deer, bear, woodchucks…"

"Anyway," continued Mac, "Ian and me came to Billy with all of these charts about physics and such trying to show Billy what the goal was and how we could get better. We're both engineers so we were analyzing our performance from that perspective. When we started out we were both pretty bad."

"So what did Billy do? I mean I don't really know what he does?" Annie asked.

"Well, it's kinda hard to explain," said Ian as he pulled the arrow out of the boar's butt. "But he never did look at any of the charts we brought. He just asked us lots of questions about our routine, how we felt when we did certain things and how that influenced our performances. Then he just told us to go out and collect data, not on our external results so much, but to slow down and pay attention to our inner results—to know how to process our results, to learn from them, to grow."

"So what happened?" Annie asked as they walked towards the smell of Pelican Stew wafting over the beach.

"Well, we're the results," said Ian as both he and Mac posed to show off their buff bodies to Annie. "What do you think? Not too shabby, huh, for a couple of middle age guys? We each lost about 20 pounds."

"And national champions to boot," exclaimed Mac.

"Impressive," said Annie, a little embarrassed. They certainly didn't fit her impression of the typical hunter.

"Well, aren't you going to ask how we did it?" Mac exclaimed.

"Well, how'd you do it?" asked Annie, playing along.

"I'm so glad you asked," Ian replied. "Billy helped us see that it's very simple, or, 'simply elegant' as Billy likes to say. As we collected our data, we discovered that we really liked field archery. We liked the feel of being in the woods, of drawing the bow, of the arrow flying through the air, of being around the other competitors. And we realized that our approach to performing the way we liked to feel was not matching up. I mean we would sometimes go out drinking the night before competitions, eat fast food, and our idea of exercise was, you know, flexing the elbow with the poof juice as our resistance." Ian and Mac demonstrated the motion for full effect.

"Poof juice?" Annie asked.

"You know, beer," said Ian.

Mac jumped in. "What Ian is trying to say is that once we committed to the internal process, we experienced this strong connection between how we felt, how we performed, and what we were doing, or weren't doing, with our bodies. We just started playing around with that stuff. We started running, eating better, and getting more rest."

"But who taught you how to do all of that stuff?" Annie asked. "Did you go to the Y or something?"

"Good God, no," Ian replied. "We taught ourselves...watch this..."

In what seemed like one motion, Ian and Mac had each notched an arrow, pulled the string back, and propelled their arrows through the sky heading toward Billy's shack. Annie had to duck out of the way, and as she looked up she saw each arrow strike the heart of a giant bear that had been placed on the roof.

"Bulls eye," exclaimed Mac, as he pump-fisted Annie. "Are ya ready for some stew?"

Annie nodded. She ran her hand over her hair just to make sure none of it had traveled with one of the arrows.

"Hey, boys and girls, step back. Annie gets the first bowl. She's our guest," said Billy, as he handed the bowl and spoon to Annie. Their hands touched for a moment and Annie felt a flash of déjà vu as well as excitement. She pulled away quickly.

Annie was famished and thankful to be first.

"I'm sorry about being a bit confrontational earlier," Annie said to Billy. "This all just seems kind of strange, you know, my case and everything."

"No problem," Billy said. "How do you feel?"

"I'm not sure…different."

"C'mon, Annie, we can eat on the deck," said Doc, motioning over to the shack. As Annie sat down, Doc went inside and turned the music down, which was followed by a large groan from the others.

"This stew is unbelievably good," said Annie. "What's in it?"

"I really don't know," said Doc. "Billy's been working on this slow cooking stew for years. He's got a garden somewhere, and buys everything else from the farmers markets. Just about everything is home grown and natural. Billy never eats anything processed. He slow cooks just about everything."

Annie didn't say much as they both devoured the stew.

"You know, I didn't go to the spa today," Annie said as she finished the last spoonful. "I told my friends that I did, but I didn't."

"Why not?" asked Doc.

"I'm not exactly sure," she replied. "I had all of these thoughts and emotions running through my head—*Game With No Name*, losing weight, my case. When I got there, I was just hanging out in the lobby. I wasn't getting a good vibe. And then I walked outside and saw this woman hitting tennis balls."

"How was that?"

"Well, I felt like it should be me hitting the tennis balls. It just looked like so much fun," Annie said as she leaned forward.

"Well, why didn't you just go hit tennis balls?"

"I don't know. I haven't played in a really long time, I'm out of shape, and you probably have to be a member or something. I just walked away and came back to the house." Annie wondered why she was telling this man she barely knew about this.

"Well, I guess the Spa isn't as attractive as all this," Doc said, as he made a sweeping motion with his hands. "What could be better than shooting arrows in boars' butts and eating stew at the shack."

Annie rocked back with laughter.

"So what's up with Billy?" Annie asked. "I mean what does he do?"

"He works on cases like yours."

"But I don't get it, why me? There are millions of people out there struggling with losing weight. How did he find out about me? Why me?"

"You're the chosen one. I don't know. You'd have to ask Billy why," Doc said. "I've learned not to ask too many questions."

"Well, let's say I let you guys work on my losing weight case." What do I have to do? How do you lose weight in six days?"

"You don't really have much choice," Doc said. "We've already started on your case."

"You have?"

"Of course. What do you think we've been doing all day? You can either let us in or resist. Your call."

Annie didn't say anything so Doc quickly followed up. "Just a warning. Don't make the mistake of getting attracted to Billy—physically, I mean."

"I'm married," Annie said, a bit too defensively.

"I know."

Obi came up with a tennis ball in his mouth, tail wagging, foaming at the mouth, begging for someone to play his game.

"His name's Obi," Doc said.

"Hi Obi," said Annie as she rubbed his nose. "Drop it," Annie commanded.

Obi obeyed.

Annie grabbed the slimy orb and gave it a toss into the sand. Obi dashed to retrieve it and was back in no time. Both Doc and Annie smiled. "Down, Obi," Doc said, and the lab reluctantly agreed.

Annie looked out towards the ocean. The fire pit was dying down, the guys on the beach had dispersed, even the boars were gone. She wondered about the bear on the roof. Billy was nowhere to be seen. The start to her relaxing vacation had been interrupted by this other world, which was strange, but seemed like fun. And Ian and Mac had given her plenty to think about.

"Honestly, Doc, you guys scare me a little. I don't know you at all. I didn't plan on this obviously."

"All I will say is just trust, Billy, he's a real doctor. I'm a doctor just not a real one."

"You mean Billy's an MD."

"Yep."

"And you're a PhD?"

"Yep."

"Wow. I wouldn't have guessed that."

"Thanks a lot."

"No, no, I mean I wouldn't have guessed Billy to be a physician."

Well, there's a lot you don't want to know, a lot you don't need to know, and a lot you'll never know about Billy Pelican. All you need to know is that we aren't here to judge you; we aren't here to change you. Everyone has a clean, unspoiled spot. Touch that spot and you lose weight. Cloak it over, try to fill it like a hole, build walls around it, and you gain weight."

"It's that simple, huh?"

Well, it's simple, but not easy," Doc said. "It's getting close to my bedtime, and I bet your friends are waking up just in time to go to bed. They'll probably want to see you." Annie was going to ask how Doc knew about her friends but she was beginning to realize that Doc and Billy knew a lot more than they were telling.

"I guess I'll sleep on all this," Annie said. "Maybe I'll see you tomorrow?"

"We're not going anywhere."

"Thanks for the stew. And thank Billy for me."

"You're welcome. And I will."

Doc grabbed the empty bowls and headed inside with Obi following close behind. As Annie walked on the path back to her house, she saw what looked like Billy sitting on an old, wooden swing on the side of the shack. She stopped for a moment to watch and then continued home.

The bear on the roof still had the two arrows sticking in its heart.

As Annie entered the house, Kate and Sam were awake and sitting on the sofa.

"There she is," said Kate. "We were just about to come outside and look for you."

"What were you doing?" asked Sam.

"Nothing much. The guys next door offered me some pelican...I mean...chicken stew. I'm sorry. I should have come and got you guys. It was really good."

"That's all right. We made a couple of sandwiches. We're still a little sluggish," said Kate, rubbing her head.

Sam was going through the text messages on her phone with a quizzical expression on her face.

"Hey, Annie," Sam said. "I'm looking at my texts and I have one from the Spa that says if I want to reschedule the appointment from today to just give them a call." Sam had used her cell number when booking the appointment for Annie.

Busted.

"Okay, guys, it's time to come clean," said Annie, as she plopped down on the couch in between her two best friends for over 30 years. "I guess it's time to tell you about my day."

Annie told most of the story, leaving out her physical attraction to Billy.

"I'm sorry I lied to you guys about the Spa but my mind was a mess," said Annie as she concluded the story.

"Oh, we don't care about that," said Kate, as she looked to Sam for reassurance. Sam nodded.

"Should we call the police? Are these guys stalking you?" asked Sam.

"No, no, nothing like that."

"You don't believe them, do you?" asked Sam.

"What do you mean?" asked Annie.

"I mean you don't think they're on this case or whatever to help you lose weight, do you?" asked Sam. "I mean, no offense, Annie, but you can't really lose much weight in six days, at least not in a healthy way. No one can."

"Well, I've tried everything else. What if these guys are for real? They seem genuine."

"You've got the hots for this Billy guy, don't you." Sam said, as she leaped off the sofa. "I would know that look anywhere."

Annie shook her head.

"Annie's got a boyfriend, Annie's got a boyfriend, Annie's got a boyfriend," Sam chanted. Kate joined in.

"Annie's got a boyfriend, Annie's got a boyfriend, Annie's got a boyfriend…"

"I do not."

"It's just like the movies. You should just have wild, passionate sex with Billy on the beach during a full moon," Sam said. "I think there's one tomorrow."

"Don't be ridiculous."

"AAAOOOOWWWWW," Sam howled.

"This is silly. I knew I shouldn't have told you guys.

AAAOOOOWWWWW," Sam howled again.

"Sam, you'll wake up our neighbors," warned Kate.

"Good, let 'em come on over and let me take a look at these so-called caseworkers," Sam retorted. "I'll give them a real case to handle."

"SAM," said both Kate and Annie.

"Okay, okay, I'm kidding…sort of," said Sam. "But you should still have sex with this man. That's would I would do."

"It's not like that," said Annie, as she thought about Sam getting her nails into Billy. She certainly couldn't compete with Sam in that arena.

"Well, what are you going to do, Annie?" Kate asked.

"I don't really want to think about it now. It's been a long day," said Annie. "I guess I'll sleep on it."

"All I know is that the beach is calling my name for tomorrow," said Sam.

"Me too," said Kate.

"Me three," said Annie. "I'm going up to bed. I'm so glad you guys are here and could have some fun at my expense. Good night."

"Good night, Annie Oakley."

"Good night, Lil Orphan Annie."

Annie thought about calling home but was too tired. She'd call tomorrow. As she was just about to drift off to sleep, she heard the beep of an incoming text and couldn't help herself:

"Go for a run on the beach, 6 am? Doc"

These guys are relentless, Annie thought. She didn't even bother worrying about how Doc got her number. She thought about her day. And then it dawned on her that no matter how bizarre it had been, she liked it. She liked watching the silly games, she liked watching the tennis player, she liked, actually loved, the stew. She liked talking with Ian and Mac. She liked trying to hit a boar's butt. She liked hanging out with her best friends. She had liked all of it. This feel excited her and scared her at the same time. The spot had been touched, had been reawakened. Deep down she knew it. What to do about it?

"Ok" Annie texted back, and set her phone alarm for 5:45 am.

"What she'd say?" asked Billy.

"Okay," replied Doc.

"Good job, Doc. That was genius planting Chrissie at the tennis courts today."

"Well, anything to get her away from that damn Spa," Doc said.

"Good night."

Doc almost said "ditto" but remembered that Billy did most of his work at night. That's when all the calls came.

Day 2
Feel

Three

Billy Pelican's White Horse Island roots ran much deeper than the fire pit hole he dug to make his locally famous Pelican Stew. Billy's great grandfather (paternal) was one of the first surfmen of the Outer Banks. Legend has it that he was a descendant of Blackbeard, who roamed the waters off the coast of North Carolina for years. Surfmen patrolled the beaches of the Outer Banks and risked their lives to save sailors and passengers of ships who were in distress. Wanting his son, Billy's grandfather, to have a safer existence, he taught him to hunt and fish. Billy's grandfather was on his way to fight the Germans when his boat received the news that the Germans had surrendered. He returned to the Outer Banks, and in the roaring 20s rich tourists sought after Billy's grandfather as the best hunting and fishing guide on the islands. Wealthy businessmen would travel the hundreds of miles from up north in the fall to hunt duck and geese that migrated to the Banks for the winter. He was also a smart businessman and a visionary. While Billy's grandfather was proprietor of the Whalehead Club—built by a wealthy businessmen as the only hunting club for both men and women—he started buying up beach front property up and down the north shore with his savings from the booming guide business. He fell in love with, and married, the only daughter of the wealthy businessman and in 1930 Billy's father was born: William Jefferson Hamilton III.

In the 1930s, 40s, and 50s, bridges were built to connect the mainland to the Banks, which dramatically increased the tourism to the islands. Property values skyrocketed after World War II and Billy's grandfather made a mint as he sold properties at exorbitant prices to the wealthy who viewed the Banks as a desirous summer residence. By the time William Jefferson Hamilton IV came along in 1961, most of the islands were growing.

But the one thing that Billy's grandfather never sold was the shack he had built on White Horse Island for his grandson. He left strict orders in his will that upon his death, the shack and the adjoining property could not be sold and were to be bequeathed to Billy. The Spa developers tried to buy the property to build a rental home for use by guests, but Billy's grandfather wouldn't budge, even after being offered exorbitant sums of money. Eventually, the developers gave up.

Billy's education began on the beaches of White Horse Island. It was during his childhood that his grandfather introduced him to the legend of the White Horses.

Annie was a little late getting down to the beach. Her alarm had felt like a sledgehammer bashing her brain. The only thing that got her out of bed was the allure of running on the beach. She had brought some running clothes and shoes just in case the move-my-body muse had struck during her week at WHI. She used to run as part of her training for tennis but after awhile kids and work pushed all of that physical activity aside. Doc's offer to run together was perfect timing. Her only fear was that she wouldn't be able to keep up.

Doc was waiting, stretching as hints of light began to appear on the horizon.

"Sorry I'm a little late," said Annie.

"No problem, my body takes a bit longer to get ready these days," Doc said.

Annie tried to do some quick arm and leg stretches and while doing so noticed that Doc was wearing the wraparound sunglasses. She wondered how he could see anything.

"I thought we could run to the pier and back," Doc said. "If we time it right we can watch the sunrise from the pier and then head back."

"That sounds wonderful," Annie said. "How far is the pier?"

"About two miles. Are you up for it?"

"As long as we go slow."

"No worries. We'll go at talking speed. But you don't have to talk if you don't want to."

In Doc's thirty-plus years of running, he rarely ran with a partner or in a group because he felt it detracted from immersing himself in the environment. There were only a handful of people he had let in to his running world.

They started out in silence focusing on getting a rhythm going and acclimating to running in sand, which was a lot different than running on roads or trails. Doc made sure he let Annie set the pace. He observed her gait and saw a couple of things that she could work on.

Annie labored the first few minutes as the motion was a shock to her heart and lungs, but soon she found the rhythm.

"So how did you meet Billy? Annie asked, when she finally caught her second wind.

"Oh, we met at a pickup basketball game that was organized at a conference we were attending on behavioral medicine. We ended up on the same team."

"Are there any games you guys don't play?" Annie commented. "Did your team win?"

"I don't really remember although I'm sure we did. I realized right away that Billy was the best player on the floor so I just fed him the ball. I found out later that he had a basketball scholarship at the University of Virginia."

"He did? Billy played at UVa?" I don't remember him. "I was born and raised in Charlottesville."

"Well, he didn't play much. This would have been the late 70s, early 80s. I guess he butted heads with the coach. I think he transferred after a couple of years and then went back to UVa for his medical degree.

Annie had so many questions about Billy but she didn't want to appear too interested based on Doc's comment last night.

They ran for a while in silence. They were both getting into the feel of the run, although it was quite a bit slower than Doc's normal pace. But it was fun for Doc, who typically pushed himself according to a preordained pace.

"So are you still in Charlottesville?" Doc broke the silence.

"Yep. Never left. I started working at the YMCA in high school and college and then just stuck around. Now I run the place."

"What do you like most about it?"

"Well, I love the members. I enjoy interacting with them, especially our older members. I just don't get to do that too much anymore."

"Why not?"

"Do you know anything about the Y?"

"A little."

"Well, there's a lot of fund raising and national programming initiatives that take a lot of planning and organizing. There's a lot of pressure to meet the financial bottom lines and we have a lot of competition."

"So where is the mind-body-spirit triangle in all of that?" Doc asked.

"Oh, well, we do wellness for our members with yoga and things like that."

"No, I meant for you."

"Oh."

While Annie pondered that one, she could see the pier jutting out into the ocean. She naturally picked up the pace a bit as she felt a rush of excitement to be so close to her first sunrise at the Outer Banks. Doc was happy to be moving a bit faster. As they made their way on to the pier, Annie saw the wondrous orange circle of fire rising up over the ocean. She moved faster, passing some early morning fishermen, finally arriving at the end of the pier. With arms raised in triumph she did a little dance until she realized Doc was watching her, and stopped.

"Don't stop on my account," said Doc.

"This is awesome," said Annie as she watched the sun make its slow ascent toward the heavens. "I wish I had the beach to run on every day."

"Yea, makes it easier, doesn't it."

"I'll say. Charlottesville's nice but not like this."

Annie felt the sweat run down her face. Felt good. "Do you run every day, Doc?"

"Pretty much. I can't run as hard as I used to though. But I still like it."

"So what are you a professor of?" asked Annie.

"Well, we're talking about it," replied Doc. "Motivation, well-being, and how they connect to health behaviors like physical activity. That's why I'm here." Doc cut right to the chase. Time was running out.

"So what do you know that can help me?" Annie asked.

"Well, it's not so much what I know but what I feel."

"What do you mean?"

"I run because it connects to how I want my life to feel."

"How do you want to feel?" asked Annie.

"Energetic, light, catalytic."

"Catalytic? What's that mean?"

"You know, I like to start things, get things going."

"I don't really know how I want to feel most of time," Annie said.

"That's why you're here, to explore your feel, to rediscover it."

"And I'll lose weight by doing that? How do I do that?

"You're doing it."

"I don't get it."

"Look, the mainstream way we go about trying to help people be healthy is totally messed up," Doc said, getting more animated.

"What do you mean?" Annie was interested for herself but also for the Y.

"Well, we spend all of this time and money trying to convince people of the benefits of exercising, eating right, managing stress, forging relationships, and so on as a means for preventing disease or obesity, thereby living longer.

"Well, what's so wrong with that?" Annie asked.

"Do you really want me to go into the woeful statistics?"

"Good point."

"It doesn't work. Most people know what they should be doing. They know what to do. But they don't do it. Look how hard you have to work just to get members at your Y? Even with your best efforts under this model, retention of your members is even more difficult so you double your efforts to attract more new members and the cycle continues."

Annie had to admit that was the truth.

"So why do so many people, including myself I hate to admit, have so much trouble doing these health behaviors even though we know they're good for us?" Annie asked.

"After all these years, the conclusion I have come to is that they are too quick to give themselves up to experts and to supposed know how because they think health is something they should possess, or something they want. Most of these people are seeking something outside of themselves and look to some expert who knows even less about them than they themselves do."

"Well, not all of them. I think you're exaggerating a little."

"Maybe a little."

"All right, doctor, let's say that's true. What do you suggest? Wellness coaching?" Annie asked.

"Oh, God, no. Wellness coaching. You can't be serious?" said Doc, using the best John McEnroe impression he could muster.

Annie was old enough to get the McEnroe imitation. "Well, we do wellness coaching at the Y," exclaimed Annie.

"That's fine. Look, I'm not here to bash coaching, but most health or wellness coaching ends up focusing on lifestyle change within *The Game* people are told to play. In other words, cope with your present lot by changing your behavior."

"I don't quite see what's wrong with that approach." Annie said.

"Well, your present lot is what's preventing you from performing these so-called healthy behaviors in the first place. People who try to lose weight or exercise or eat right without knowing how they want to feel just succumb to the techniques of the day; they give themselves up to the experts, and fail miserably because of it. They attempt to do expert-driven,

health-related behaviors in an attempt to cope with their present life experiences rather than connecting health-related behaviors to something deep
inside them that enhances or transforms their life experiences—the feel of
living."

"Aren't you just describing wellness? Annie asked.

"I don't think so. Wellness is just health disguised as something else to
get you to practice techniques taught by more experts working within a
fragmented, biomedical model. I mean seriously why did you decide to run
with me this morning? Were you thinking about protecting yourself from
cardiovascular disease, cancer, or diabetes? Your spirituality? Your feelings?
Or, heaven forbid, bringing balance to your life?"

"Not really," Annie replied. "I guess I was curious and thought it might
be fun."

"Exactly. And was it?"

"Yes, it was…until now."

"OMG. You are so right. I've just been ranting," said Doc. "I'm sure I
spoiled the sunrise. I'm so sorry. I'll shut up now." Doc could have kicked
himself for getting on the soapbox. Stupid.

Annie and Doc looked out towards the ocean. Annie spotted a pod of
pelicans gliding on top of the waves. There was just something mesmer-
izing about pelicans in flight. Doc could sense that Annie was back in the
moment. He let her watch them till they were out of sight.

"Well, do you want to head back?" Doc asked. "How do you feel?"

"I'm good. I can jog another two miles." Annie replied.

The return trip was quieter, with Doc afraid to say too much and Annie
struggling with the rhythm. She kept wondering about *feel*. What a strange
word, she thought.

Near the end, Doc said: "Let's stop, take our shoes off, and sprint to the
end. It's only about 100 yards."

"I'm way ahead of you," said Annie as she plopped her shoes and socks
off, put them in her hands and took off. Doc struggled with double knots
he always tied and got a late start. Annie was faster than Doc thought so he
really had to kick it in gear to catch her and then let her win by the length
of a pelican's beak.

Annie broke into the Rocky theme song and raised her hands high again using her shoes and socks as boxing gloves. Then they both dropped to the sand and made sand angels.

"So what game are you guys playing?" a voice asked that seemed to come right out of the waves. Annie, shading her eyes from the sun, made out Billy's gigantic body coming towards them. "We are playing the sand angels-boxing gloves-running game," said Annie.

"Well, that's a pretty lame title," said Billy. "But at least you're playing."

Annie and Doc sat up, their bodies covered in sand.

"What are you doing out here so early, Doctor Pelican?" Annie asked.

"Well, this is pretty much the best time to come out to body surf before the beach gets full of non pelicans," Billy replied.

"I agree," Annie said. "Doc and I just ran to the pier and back. Well, it was probably a jog for Doc, but I was running. Felt great."

"Sounds good. I saw you running, I mean jogging, back."

Billy reached out his hand to help Annie up. Annie locked her hand with Billy's as he pulled her upright. Again, she couldn't help but notice the size of Billy's hand, and she felt that same rush of familiarity and excitement as the previous night. Billy ignored Doc's outstretched hand.

"Thanks a lot," Doc said, as he worked himself to his feet.

Billy got right into it turning to Annie. "I noticed that when you were running you were hunched over a little. Are you aware that you do that?"

"No, what, I hunch over?" Annie looked over at Doc, who nodded.

"Yea, I've also noticed it when you walk too. Do you have back problems?"

"Well, actually, I have had some lower back pain the last few years. I've tried a little physical therapy but it hasn't helped much. "

"It's probably from hunching over or slouching. Why do you slouch?"

"I...I...I'm not sure," Annie stammered. She hadn't expected the inquisition. "I wasn't really aware that I was doing it."

"Well, how we carry ourselves is usually indicative of how we feel about ourselves. You kind of carry yourself like you're in mourning or a little bit sad. It shows up in your walking and running. I bet your house is a little sad too."

"I don't feel that way," Annie stated emphatically.

"Now who's lying," Billy replied.

"I really don't have to stand here and take this from you, a perfect stranger I barely know." Annie said, visibly upset.

"I'm not here to judge you. I'm just making an observation."

After Doc had worked with Billy awhile, he began stuffing tissues in his pocket because invariably there was some crying. Unfortunately, he didn't have access to any in the middle of the beach.

Silence, except for the waves. Billy was used to it. Doc hated it but he had learned the hard way that the silence was essential to the process.

Doc guessed that Annie might just walk away—but she didn't. She just stood there with her head down.

Billy grabbed a small stone and stick. In the sand near Annie's feet he placed the stone and then drew several circles around it:

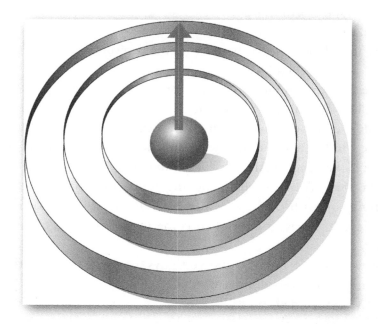

Billy started in: "The stone is you, it's your spot, that clean, unspoiled spot inside that is unique to each of us. Over time many people try to protect the spot by building walls around it. This doesn't work, of course, and after awhile people are so weighed down by the walls that they've forgotten about their spot, or can't reach it. Without touching that spot, growing it, nurturing it, life becomes about living within the walls, and you no longer experience those moments of silence, of stillness; those moments when you feel weightless."

After a few seconds, Annie looked up from the figure Billy had drawn in the sand. Her eyes were red. Doc knew that feeling.

"Doc was right. You are an asshole." Annie said, but she was smiling even as she wiped away the tears with her fingers. "I haven't felt those moments that you described in quite awhile.

"When have you felt them?"

"Well, since I've been here I've had a few of those moments. Like sprinting there at the end of my run. I felt free, like it was me. Of course, I know I'll be sore tomorrow."

"But it was worth it, right?"

"Yea, sure."

Just then Doc saw two women heading toward them. "I think we've got company," warned Doc.

Kate and Sam sauntered up with Sam leading the charge.

"Hello, I'm Sam, and this is Kate," she said, sizing up Billy and Doc as she made the introductions. "You must be the guys next door. We saw you from the window and thought we'd come down and see what's going on."

Sam looked over at Annie. "Everything okay, honey?"

"Yea, yea," Annie replied, looking down to avoid eye contact. "I went for a run with Doc. We've just been discussing, uh, posture, if you can believe it. I was just about to come in and make you guys a killer breakfast."

"So what's this about a case you guys are working on with Annie," asked Sam, never one to mince words.

"SAM," exclaimed Annie.

"What's this in the sand?" asked Kate, who was a little more curious than Sam.

Doc started in: "Well, that stone is your spot—"

"My spot…my spot," interjected Sam. "What are you guys perverts or something? C'mon, Annie, let's go," as she grabbed Annie's arm.

The three women headed back to the house.

"HEY, ANNIE, IF YOU WANT TO LEARN HOW TO BODY SURF, MEET ME HERE TOMORROW MORNING," Billy yelled.

Without looking back, Annie raised the arm that wasn't in Sam's vice grip and gave a thumb's up.

*D*oc placed his sunglasses on the sand, waded out in the water, and then dove in to wash the sand from his body. Billy was sitting in the sand waiting for him as he got out of the water.

"How was the run?" Billy asked.

"Good. I probably talked a bit too much on the pier, but at least I didn't make her cry. Good grief."

"You know the crying is just an emotional reaction when like versus want collide. She's starting to open up to the like again."

"I hadn't thought about the posture and overweight connection," Doc said, as he put on his sunglasses to protect his eyes. "But I guess if you're weighed down by want, you're going to slouch."

"Well, people are overweight because want is an unnatural way of doing things. It won't matter what wellness or positive psychology programs or coaching you fling at them," said Billy. They're still addressing the symptoms, not the core issues."

"Do you think Sam is going to be a problem?" Doc asked.

"Could be. I might have to do something."

"Like what?"

"I have a couple of ideas."

Billy and Doc both felt that Annie had made some progress but there was a long way to go to weightlessness. Sam was getting in the way.

"You know why I like pelicans so much?" asked Billy.

"No, why?"

"See those pelicans out there?" Billy asked as he pointed in their direction so Doc could see them.

"The whole health and fitness industry has it all wrong. Charles Lindberg said: 'Building an airplane is easier than the evolutionary process of the flight of a bird. I'd rather be around birds.' Building planes is fake, an unnatural creation. No offense to the Wright brothers. Birds are natural. That's why pelicans look so beautiful in flight. They're not trying to change; they're just being themselves. Health and fitness is trying to build planes instead of helping people touch and feel what comes naturally to them."

"I get that," Doc said. "I just find it an interesting paradox that if it's so natural why so few people do it.

"They're too busy building planes," Billy replied.

Doc felt something touch his back. He turned to see that it was Obi.

"Obi," Doc cried out with enthusiasm. "Good to see you buddy." He grabbed the stick that Billy had used to draw the circular walls and heaved it in the ocean. Both Obi and Billy dashed in after it. Obi beat Billy to the punch, fetched the stick, and carried it back to Doc.

Billy stayed in the water, preparing for the next round of body surfing.

Doc watched as the incoming waves washed away the walls around the stone and hoped that Annie could do the same.

Kate and Sam were on the deck off the kitchen—probably talking about Doc and Billy. Annie felt it as she made breakfast. The experience of the run on the beach, the sunrise, even the crying, had touched her. She felt alive—some deep inner sense of herself had been awakened.

She scrambled the eggs with a vengeance and cut up the strawberries with keen precision. She prepared the Bloody Marys with a passion that had been missing in her life for quite some time. She reminded herself to stand up straight. Stay tall, be strong, she thought. She had this renewed energy, unsure of the source.

She carried the plates full of food out to Kate and Sam. "Bloody Marys coming up," as she dashed back into the kitchen.

"This looks great, Annie." Said Kate.

"Fabulous," said Sam.

"Here's to White Horse Island and friendship," said Annie as she raised her glass.

"To friendship," said Kate.

"To wild sex," said Sam.

"SAM," said Kate and Annie together.

"Dig in," said Annie.

Annie's hunger was voracious. Everything seemed to have a new taste, like she was eating for the first time.

"So what happened down by the water?" asked Sam. "Were they taking you through some kind of ritual with that stone. Are they part of a cult or something?"

"No, don't be silly," replied Annie. "I just took a run on the beach with Doc, then Billy said I had bad posture and called me a liar. That's when you guys showed up."

"The nerve of that guy," said Sam.

"A liar? What do you mean?" asked Kate.

"Well, mostly lying to myself...I think," said Annie. "Billy said that my bad posture indicated that I was sad."

"I said I didn't feel that way, and that's when he called me a liar. He was just using the stone to make his case."

"Well, do you feel sad?" asked Sam as she downed her Bloody Mary.

"I don't know but I do know the last few years I haven't really felt myself, like something's missing. I started crying when I was looking at some of our old pictures in my room. I noticed that my smile was huge back in high school. I wondered where my smile went and I just started balling."

"You brought pictures with you?" asked Sam.

"Yes."

"Well go get them girl. I've got to see these," said Sam.

Annie dashed upstairs and was back in moments, shoebox in tow. Sam had replenished the empty glasses.

They grabbed the pictures—tennis, prom, hanging out—like they were free money.

"I was so skinny," said Sam.

"You still are," said Kate, shaking her head. "Wow, Annie, you do have a great smile."

"Man, we look good," said Sam.

Annie was glad she had brought the pictures. They spent a few hours reminiscing as each picture sparked a story about something. They were full of promise back then. Annie couldn't get her coach's words out of her head: "Never lose that smile." Somewhere along the way she had lost it. Since her arrival at White Horse Island, she had found it again. And as crazy as it seemed, just thinking of Doc and Billy made her smile.

"What are you smiling about, Annie Oakley?" asked Kate, interrupting her thoughts.

"Oh, nothing. It's just nice to feel something that's right about me, that's right about us. Let's hit the beach."

Four

ANNIE PLAYS FRIZWIFF

*T*he beach was starting to fill up but the three women found plenty of space to set up behind the house. Once settled in on the towels, they sat looking out to the ocean.

"This is beautiful," said Annie.

"Glorious," said Kate.

"Who wants a beer?" said Sam as she reached into the cooler.

"To life-long friendship and fun," Annie said, as they toasted.

Annie couldn't get the thoughts of the stone and the walls that Billy drew around it out of her mind. Her conversations with Doc and Ian and Mac rose up in her consciousness. Her mind was full of wonder and doubt about it all.

"So what are you thinking about?" Kate asked, picking up on Annie's thoughts.

"Well, I'm sitting here wondering about my spot, you know the stone in the sand."

"What do you mean?" asked Kate.

"Well, when I was making you guys breakfast, I had all of this energy. I'm not sure where it was coming from. Before I arrived here I felt like I've been going through the motions. Making breakfast I felt different."

"Well, you are on vacation," suggested Sam.

"But I don't think that's it," Annie said. "I feel different, like something is growing inside me. It's weird. I can't explain it."

"I think those guys are crackpots," said Sam. "You know, like the Secret. Remember that? Laws of attraction and all of that malarkey."

"Maybe. But Billy's an MD…"

"Hey, MDs can be crackpots too," Sam reminded Annie. "Where'd he get his degree Moron Medical School?"

"Actually, he got it at UVa," Annie replied.

"OOOOOHHHHH, impressive," Sam chided. "I take it back."

"Look, Annie, if you feel like these guys can be trusted then just go with it, said Kate. "See what happens. I mean nothing bad has happened to you so far, has it?" Kate was always the adventurous one.

"Well, no…but…"

"Then just see what happens," Kate advised, looking to Sam for approval.

"Yeah, sure, what the heck," said Sam. "But I would still screw Billy just for fun."

Annie's sunbathing slumber was interrupted by a sense that something was touching her legs. She swatted at whatever it was with her hand. But the sensation returned moments later. As she turned her head to look back and opened her eyes, she spotted a big, yellow creature and jumped off the towel. Now that she was awake, Annie realized it was Obi. He had been trying to retrieve a wiffleball that somehow had come to rest between her thighs.

"Obi, my gosh, you scared me," Annie said, as Obi wagged his tail and scooped up the ball in his mouth. Annie recognized Doc walking towards her.

"Sorry about that," said Doc. "Looks like your friends are truly out to lunch," pointing to Kate and Sam who were dead to the world.

"Yea, they had a few beers on top of some Bloody Marys. I was wise enough to stop."

"Well, do you want to join our game?" Doc asked.

"What crazy name game are you guys playing this time?" Annie asked.

"Not sure exactly. I think we call it *Frizwiff*. You can be on my team."

Annie looked over at Kate and Sam. They were going to be out for awhile.

"What the heck. I'm in," Annie said. Her positive reply surprised her.

As they walked toward the action, Doc yelled out, "OKAY, EVERYONE, THIS IS ANNIE. SHE'S ON MY TEAM."

"HI ANNIE," Everyone yelled out in unison.

"Okay, Annie, you're up."

"What do I do?" Annie asked.

"Oh, well, you throw this Frisbee, keeping it within the fair lines, and then run the bases like baseball," Doc said as he pointed to the three plastic, orange-colored bases, which looked rather far apart.

"That's it?"

"Oh, if anyone on the other team catches the disc, the other team's players can throw the wiffleball at you or hit you with the wifflebat while you're running. If the ball or bat touch you, you're out. They can't throw the bat or ball at you if the Frisbee touches the ground anywhere past the three bases. They can only get you out then by hitting you with the Frisbee. Oh, and you have to keep running until you're either out or reach home.

"They can hit me with the bat?" Annie asked. "Won't that hurt?"

"I guess it could. Just try to dodge the bat," Doc said, as he rubbed the welt on his arm. "Are you ready?" Doc asked, as he handed Annie the Frisbee.

"I guess," Annie answered, stepping up to the plate.

Annie looked out to the field and saw bodies spread out over the entire field. She felt the wind whipping in from the ocean.

She tried to remember how she used to throw the Frisbee with her brother on summer days when they had nothing else to do. After a few practice swings, she let it fly and started running her fastest to first.

She saw the disc curve in the wind and land outside the first base line.

"FOUL," Doc yelled, as he caught the Frisbee tossed back in by one of the fielders.

Annie jogged back. She was already winded and her legs were fatigued from the morning jog with Doc.

"Not bad," Doc said. "Try to keep it fair this time. You're only allowed one foul throw."

Annie nodded. She adjusted her stance, like she was getting ready to return serve in the ad court. This time she angled the disc a bit so it would cut into the wind. Surprisingly, the disc soared into the air out towards centerfield as Annie ran. As she rounded first, she saw one of the guys dive for the disc and somehow catch it with his fingertips as he smashed head first into the sand. He raised the disc high to indicate a catch. As Annie neared second, she now realized that she was in danger of being smacked by the ball or bat. She felt fear, cold-blooded fear. She rounded second and looked back just in time to see the ball thrown by the second baseman heading toward her butt. She jumped high enough to have the ball whistle through her legs missing her by inches and roll toward the third baseman who held his bat like a knight would hold his sword just before slaying the dragon. Obi came to the rescue. Running from home to retrieve what he thought was *his* ball, Obi, the ball, and Annie arrived at third base at the same time. Obi dashed in to retrieve the ball knocking over the bewildered third baseman, as the bat flew from his hands. This freed the path for Annie who touched third base and rounded for home. Gasping for breath, she could see home plate and believed she was home free.

With just a few steps to go to score a run for her team, Annie heard something whistling toward her. As she turned her head to the sound, the flying disc hammered into her forehead, forcing her to lose her balance and fall backwards toward home plate. As Annie was falling, she somehow reached out with her hand to touch home plate just before she slumped to the sand and blacked out.

—⟜

*A*nnie felt Billy hold her and kiss her lips. She felt alive. Her body ached for him. She wanted to touch him, to love him, to care for him. She reached for him…

"Hey, she's coming around, she's moving her arms like she's hugging someone."

"Annie, Annie, can you hear me?"

"Give her some room. Let her breathe."

"Obi, stop licking her face."

As Annie came back to consciousness and opened her eyes, she noticed her arms in the air and quickly dropped them to her side. Her face flushed.

"Wow, you had us a little worried there Annie," said Doc. "DJ, give her the water bottle."

"Do you think it's a concussion?" one of the players asked.

"I'm not sure. We'll have to ask Billy," Doc said.

"No, no, I'm fine," said Annie, who did not want to see Billy at the moment. Annie sat up and took the water offered by DJ. "I just blacked out for a minute. What happened?"

"You don't remember?" DJ asked.

"Well, I remember running home and then being hit by something."

"I'm so sorry," DJ said. "I hit you in the head with the disc."

Annie looked up at DJ and recognized him as the player who caught her throw with a dive. "You hit me in the head from centerfield with the Frisbee?" Annie asked. "That's impossible."

"Well, typically it would be," said Doc, "but this is DJ Sweeney, the Most Valuable Player at the Ultimate World Games three years in a row."

"You mean as in Ultimate Frisbee?"

"Yea. It's called Ultimate at the higher levels of competition," DJ said. "Are you okay?"

"Yea, I think so. What are you doing here?" Annie asked.

"Billy called me, you know, to help with the case and all."

"Of course he did," mumbled Annie as Doc and DJ helped her to her feet.

"Well, the good news is that you touched home before you hit the sand," Doc said. "Your run broke the tie so our team won. Game over."

"Yeah, way to go Annie. What a run," said a woman who slapped her on the back.

"Uh…Thanks," Annie said, recognizing her as the woman who was hitting tennis balls yesterday.

"No hard feelings," DJ said as he extended his hand.

Annie and DJ shook hands. "No, no, it was fun. Great catch and throw by the way," Annie said. Turning to Doc: "You neglected to tell me that they could also hit me with the Frisbee *after* a catch," Annie said.

"I thought I mentioned that…well, that's a relatively new rule," said Doc. "Maybe I forgot. You sure you don't want Billy to take a look at you?" Doc asked.

"I'm sure. I should probably go see if Kate and Sam are awake. We talked about shopping and dinner in town this evening."

Doc looked disappointed upon hearing this news, which Annie picked up on.

"Why, did you have more games in mind that include blows to the head?" Annie asked.

Doc liked the sarcasm but ignored it.

"Well, I was just thinking that I could help you and your friends create a game that all of you might want to play together," said Doc.

"I'll need to think about that," said Annie, as she touched the bump on her forehead. "I don't want to put my friends' lives in danger. It's not their case."

Each player came up to Annie and fist bumped her. They seemed genuinely concerned about her well-being. The tennis woman gave her a hug.

As she walked toward her friends, she saw the Frisbee fly by her with Obi running after it. He timed his leap perfectly and snatched it out of the air.

Even the dog's got some game, thought Annie. Who are these guys?

"YOU MIGHT WANT TO ICE THAT BUMP," Doc yelled after her.

Annie waved without looking back.

*B*ack at the house, Kate was grabbing cubes of ice from the freezer and filling a plastic bag full. On the sofa, Sam was giving Annie the third degree.

"I don't get it. How can any of this be helping you lose weight? I mean this champion Frisbee dude slams your head with a Hurculean fling. Seriously? Why can't they just throw the Frisbee like normal people on the beach or play wiffleball."

"Well, I guess then it wouldn't be *The Game With No Name*," Annie replied.

Kate placed the bag gently on Annie's forehead as Annie leaned her head back against the back of the sofa.

"Was it fun though?" asked Kate. "I mean before you got hit by the head-seeking missile."

"I didn't get to play very long but, yes, it was fun. I threw the Frisbee, ran around the bases, and dodged a wiffleball. Now that I think about it, it was hilarious when Obi knocked down the third baseman."

Annie started laughing out loud but that hurt her head so she stopped.

"When I was out, I dreamed that Billy Pelican kissed me," Annie blurted out.

Kate and Sam looked at each other. Annie wasn't one to divulge personal information unless it was poked or probed or prodded out of her.

"Annie Jackson, you wild woman," said Sam. "All right, that's what I'm talking about. Is there a full moon tonight? You should have shack sex with the real doctor, you know like in that one movie when Jeff Bridges and Rachel Ward are on that island."

"Annie, don't listen to crazy, Sam," said Kate. "Dreams can be interpreted in so many different ways."

"Don't listen to goody two-shoes over there," said Sam. "If you've got the hots for someone, you've got the hots. Go with it."

Doc warned me not to act on my physical attraction to Billy," Annie said.

"Why not?" asked Sam.

"I don't know."

"Well, forget that fake doc," said Sam. "Professors are always screwing their students. Mine did! What does he know? I think it would be the best thing for you."

Kate tried to shift the conversation: "I think we should forget about all of this sex stuff and games and head into town for shopping and dinner. Are you up for it, Annie?"

"I think so," Annie said, as she removed the ice bag from her forehead and handed it to Kate. "I don't know how much fun sex would be right now anyway with this thing on my forehead. And I'm not going to have sex with Billy Pelican anyway."

"Trust me, a bump on the forehead would not get in the way of good sex," said Sam.

Annie smiled as she headed up the stairs to get ready for a relaxing night out with the girls.

Five

SERENITY NOW

*B*illy watched the three women get in the car to drive the five miles on White Horse Road into town. He knew they were going to shop and eat. That's what everyone did. He hoped Harry would do his job tonight.

Annie, Kate, and Sam were like most people who vacationed at White Horse Island: they had no idea of the history of WHI. They knew of clothing stores, Starbucks, and personal watercraft. They didn't really know the island. Billy knew that at a deeper level, this type of approach to vacationing served as a metaphor for how most people were living their lives. People distracted themselves by shopping, raising kids, working, taking vacations—and then at some point would say to themselves: "I did what I was supposed to do, it doesn't feel how I thought it would, I don't know what to do about it." That's when Billy got the calls.

Billy liked Doc because he at least recognized the folly of the mainstream mindset driven by experts and techniques. Doc was the one who realized early on that people's physical activity and what and how they ate were driven by an inner process. The more disconnected people were from touching, feeling, playing with that unspoiled spot deep inside them, the more unnatural their behavior, which led to a quality of life that was far from optimal. Doc had been interested in studying if the process could be reversed—by rediscovering and being themselves, would people move their bodies more and eat better as a natural process connected to what they liked? Billy didn't care much for the research angle that Doc took but there wasn't much he could do about it. Billy already knew that Doc would find a connection, and so what? Academics wouldn't care. They were so focused on health behavior change by targeting thoughts and feelings that nothing Doc could write or present would change their minds. Things weren't going to change through academia and research. The medical paradigm—the one that Billy fled—was so big and twisted that it ate Doc alive. Then he got sick.

Annie's case was Doc's chance to experiment and give him a renewed chance to be himself. Billy owed Doc that for believing in him when everyone else had cast him aside.

As the sun began to set on the sound, Billy thought of the White Horses. It was the White Horses that had led him to Annie. Since his return to White Horse Island, Billy had rediscovered the magic of the White Horses uncovered by his grandfather. The White Horses called to Billy and he listened. Then he called them.

Annie parked the car near the town park. Most of the shops were clustered within a ½ mile stretch on the Currituck Sound side for easy access. A walking path along the White Horse Road or Highway 12 made getting around to all the shops that much easier. As they walked, Annie made a conscious attempt to keep her back straight, to stay tall. She found if she concentrated on the balls of her feet, rather than her heels, that she had a bit more spring in her step. This made her feel lighter as she kept wondering about her feel. She avoided trying on too many clothes as this forced her to look in the mirror and she didn't really like what she saw, not to mention having to view the lump protruding from her forehead.

As the shopping progressed, Annie was just not getting that same adrenaline rush that she typically got when looking at and trying on clothes. While Sam and Kate tried on multiple outfits, Annie's mind kept drifting to the events of the past few days. Except for the muscle soreness and the bump, she felt better. But why? Billy and Doc hadn't put her on any kind of program and she wasn't following any diet plan. She had more energy and her smile was back. Sam would say it's because she was on vacation. But she certainly wasn't losing any weight. So what was the point?

"Annie…Annie, did you hear me?" Kate asked. "What do you think of this outfit?"

"Oh, yeah, very nice," Annie said, trying to look interested.

"Everything, all right?" asked Kate. "You seem a little distracted."

"No, I'm fine. Must be the bump. Plus, I'm famished. Let's finish up and find a good place for dinner."

"Okay, I'll find Sam, and we'll check out."

Walking around the town park, Annie spotted *The White Horse Bar and Grill* across the street. The place was difficult to see hidden by olive trees and the fact that the house was so small. A faded sign out front said: "Best eats in oldest house in White Horse."

"That's got to be good," said Annie, and the three women ventured inside for what turned out to be the best restaurant meal any of the women had eaten in a long, long time.

"That was great," Annie said. "Almost as good as the Pelican Stew that Billy makes. Why can't Charlottesville have a place like that?"

"Well, then Charlottesville would be in White Horse," Kate said.

The food and wine had given the women that post-dinner hangover feeling where everything slows down and you feel content, that everything is right with the world. They got a little disoriented and just walked around White Horse enjoying the peace and quiet of the night. Things were closing up in the town of White Horse. As they meandered towards the car, the only shop still open, *The White Horse Surf Shop*, whose blinking "Open" neon light was barely visible, intrigued Sam.

"Hey guys let's go in, I've never been in a surf shop before," Sam said.

Kate and Annie peered in the window. The place was old, weathered.

"I don't know, the place seems kind of run down," Kate said.

"Oh, c'mon. Where's that adventurous spirit of yours, Kate," said Sam.

Sam bolted inside before her friends could stop her, and they begrudgingly followed.

Littered throughout the store were longboards, softboards, paddle boards, body boards, and skimboards, with no particular sense of organization.

"How does this place stay in business?" whispered Kate to Annie.

"I don't know. I've never seen anything like it." Annie whispered back. "And the odor. Do you smell that? It smells like something died."

Sam stepped up on one of the longboards lying on the floor. "Hey, look at me, I'm like that actress playing Gidget in that one movie," Sam said as she attempted to look like a surfer, exaggerating the moves.

"You mean Sandra Lee in the 1959 classic, *Gidget*," said a low voice from somewhere in the back of the store, startling the women and causing Sam to lose her footing and fall off the board.

The man had mysteriously appeared from a back room, partially hidden by the chaotic arrangement of the surfboards. He had long silver hair, held together loosely by a ponytail in the back that hung over his eyes. His movie star features were weathered by age, sun, and wind. Wearing shorts, sandals, and a sleeveless t-shirt, his broad shoulders stood out like the heads on Mt. Rushmore. Annie immediately thought swimmer. She had been around the Y long enough to recognize the body type. His posture was perfect.

The man leaned over and offered a hand to Sam, who, mesmerized by the man's looks, mindlessly offered up her hand. He pulled her up close. "Hello, surf dudette, Harry Hopkins, proprietor of the White Horse Surf Shop. How may I be of service to you?"

Sam, still spellbound, had no quick retort. "Uh…uh…we just wanted to look around."

Annie couldn't believe the man's voice. It was intoxicating. Fear had turned to brain freeze.

"Well, by all means, look all you want. I'm not used to such good-looking tourists coming in. We're pretty hard core here, I mean, you know, with surfing. Not like those new dang shops where they sell skates and hats and clothes. Surf shops my ass. When I was growing up here, we didn't have any of that crap."

Annie came to her senses. "Oh, well, we were just getting ready to leave."

"Now, Annie, we're in no rush," said Sam, who couldn't take her eyes off of Harry. "Do you give surfing lessons?"

"Sure do. I'll tell you what. I'll give you ladies a discount. Annie and Kate shook their heads. Surfing was not on their bucket list.

"I will take you up on that offer," said Sam. "When can you do it?"

"Well, morning's best time to go," said Harry. "How about eight? Meet me here."

"Deal," as Sam extended her hand to close the deal.

Instead of shaking Sam's hand, Harry caressed it from underneath and lifted it up to his lips for a gentle kiss. "I look forward to it, Mrs…?"

"*Miss* Pennington, Sam Pennington."

"Lovely name. I will see you, pretty lady, in the morning."

Annie and Kate moved over to Sam to begin nudging her out of the store, all the while smiling at Harry. They had to pry Sam's hand from Harry's.

"Let me help you ladies to the door," said Harry, as he kicked some of the surfing paraphernalia out of the way to create a walking path.

As Harry reached the door, he stopped and abruptly turned to face them.

"I'll tell you what, since you seem like lovely ladies, I'll let you take any of these bags of herbal blend incense here…on the house," said Harry, as he pointed to an array of funky looking bags hanging together near the door.

"That sounds interesting," said Sam, who still had her eyes locked on Harry.

"Oh, we don't smoke pot, Harry," said Annie, who knew all about this stuff from her son, Dylan.

"It's not pot. It's herbal blend incense. Totally legal," said Harry.

"Yes, Annie, it's herbal blend incense. Let's try some," said Sam, who was already acting like she was drugged.

"I thought all of that was banned by the Feds just this year," said Annie.

"It was, but they're always coming up with new stuff that's not on the banned list. You should just give it a try. It will relax you. You seem a little uptight," said Harry.

"Well, I'm not used to perfect strangers offering to sell me some pot," Annie fired back. "I think we'd better leave." Annie and Kate veered around Harry and headed outside.

"Still on for tomorrow, Sam?" asked Harry, as he placed a pack of rolling papers in her hand.

"I wouldn't miss it for the world," said Sam. Just before she reached the door, she grabbed a bag of *Serenity Now*, stuffed it in her purse, and gave Harry a wink.

"Well, that was interesting," said Kate as they headed to the car.

"Are you really going to let that guy give you surfing lessons, Sam?" asked Annie.

"Sure, why not? He seems cool to me. Dreamy, wouldn't you say?" Sam said. Annie didn't say anything, but she had to admit, Harry was cool.

As soon as the women entered the house, Sam pulled them over to the sofa and pulled out the bag of synthetic pot from her purse like a magician would pull a rabbit out of the hat.

"Sam Pennington, what did you do?" demanded Kate.

"Oh, c'mon, Kate. You weren't always such a goody two-shoes," said Sam. "I remember those days when we would get stoned and sit on the Lawn goofing on all the nerds who walked by. And, Annie, didn't you say Dylan got caught smoking pot? Maybe we should try it and see what the attraction is?"

"Nice try, Sam. I never smoked a lot of pot till I was in college. Dylan's a freshman in high school. When I was in high school, trying pot never entered my mind until graduation night," Annie countered.

"Well, I'm going to try it. We're on vacation. This stuff is perfectly legal," Sam declared.

"I don't know, I've heard the synthetic marijuana is more dangerous," said Kate.

"We'll just take a few puffs. C'mon, live a little," Sam said.

Annie remembered those same lines that got her to smoke pot in college. She shook her head. "I don't think so."

Annie watched in disbelief as Sam took out the papers, placed the herbal incense in the paper, and rolled a joint. It did look enticing. Just looking at the joint took her back to more carefree, happier times. Annie longed for those days when the only responsibility she had was going to classes. How did my life become weighed down with so much responsibility? she wondered.

"Serenity now," said Sam, as she posed in meditative fashion.

Kate and Annie couldn't help but laugh.

"You're crazy," said Kate.

"Yes, I am," said Sam. "Tonight *Serenity Now*. Tomorrow Harry Hopkins."

Sam scooted off the sofa and dashed into the kitchen to find some matches. She ran back in shaking the box like it was a Maraca.

"Okay, ladies, let's see what all the fuss is about," said Sam as she lit the joint. "Let's see if I remember how to do this."

Kate and Annie watched as Sam actually inhaled and took a long puff on the joint. She held it in for a few seconds and then exhaled, handing the joint to Kate, who looked to Annie for her approval. Annie shrugged. While Kate took a puff, Annie watched Sam go into a coughing fit. Kate passed the joint over to Annie who hesitated and then took a puff. She purposefully inhaled less strenuously than Sam, exhaled quickly, and placed the joint on the coffee table. Sam snatched it and took another long hit. Kate and Annie passed.

A few seconds later all three rushed to the kitchen for water.

"My mouth feels like an inferno," said Kate.

"My throat is in hell," said Annie. "Get rid of that thing," pointing to the joint still in Sam's hand.

"Ick, I can't believe we used to smoke stuff like this," said Sam as she doused the joint under the running water and then flushed it down the garbage disposal.

"Well, that certainly wasn't the pot that I remember," said Kate. "How does anyone smoke that shit?"

As they walked back to the sofa, a bell rang out.

"THE COPS," yelled Sam, "IT'S THE COPS."

"Shhh, Sam," said Annie. "It's just the doorbell."

"Don't answer it, don't answer it," begged Sam. "Ohhh, I'm feeling dizzy." As Sam began to lose her balance, Kate and Annie caught her and placed her gently on the sofa.

The doorbell rang again.

"We'd better see who it is, Annie," said Kate.

Annie and Kate tidied up the pot mess and Annie walked to the door. Through the peephole she recognized Doc, without his sunglasses. She opened the door a smidge.

"Hi Annie," Doc said. "I was just checking on your forehead, and I thought, if you guys weren't too tired, I could take you through *The Game With No Name* to show you how it's done."

"Thanks, Doc. My bump is fine," said Annie, "but I'm not sure right now is the best time for the game thing. We're a little tired."

"Okay," said Doc. "You can still do the body surfing with Billy in the morning?"

"Sure," replied Annie. As she was just about to close the door, it opened up wide to reveal Sam. Annie looked back at Kate. Kate shrugged.

"Well, good ole, Doc," said Sam, who was definitely feeling the effects of *Serenity Now*, which seemed to be a misnomer. "C'mon in. Where's your big friend?"

"Oh, he's just taking some calls," said Doc, as he entered the foyer. "What's that smell?"

"Well, if you must know, being the great caseworker that you are, your casee here, just smoked pot," said Sam defiantly. "If she gets the munchies, that's not going to help her lose weight, is it? Ohhh, I'm feeling dizzy again." This time Annie and Doc caught Sam and led her back to sofa.

Annie was feeling a little lightheaded and nauseous as well so she sat down next to Kate. She then explained the entire pot-smoking incident to Doc.

"Well, synthetic pot is a little stronger than the old-fashioned stuff," said Doc, as he looked at Sam. "But the high doesn't last as long and people typically don't get the munchies."

"Thank you, Mr. Expert," said Sam.

"I'm no expert. I just remember reading a paper one of my students wrote on the topic for a class assignment."

"SKUNK, SKUNK," Sam cried out, as she jumped off the sofa and ran up the stairs. Annie quickly followed her.

"DON'T LET IT SPRAY ME, DON'T LET IT SPRAY ME..." Kate and Doc looked at each other and burst out laughing. They heard lots of running and shouting upstairs for a few minutes and then silence.

A few minutes later they saw Annie coming down the stairs.

"She finally just crashed on my bed," said Annie. "Wow."

"I probably should have mentioned that paranoia is worse with the synthetic stuff," Doc said, "although it does smell as bad as a skunk in here."

This time it was Annie and Kate's turn to laugh.

"How come you guys don't seem as bad?" asked Doc.

"Well, Kate and I just took little puffs," Annie said as she demonstrated. "We didn't inhale like we were trying to set the holding-my-breath-underwater record the way Sam did."

"Smart," Doc said.

Silence.

"You're not leaving till we do this game thing, are you?" asked Annie.

Doc shrugged.

"Okay, Doctor White Horse, how do we play?"

Doc rubbed his hands together. He loved this stuff.

—◠—

"Do you need any water or anything before we get started?" Doc asked. "No, we're good," Kate said.

"It's really quite simple," Doc said. "I usually like more than two people in a group but I don't think Miss paranoia upstairs will be joining us. You'll just have to wing it a bit and think about what Sam might like."

"Okay," said Annie. Both Kate and Annie leaned forward, eager to begin.

"In *The Game With No Name*, it's not so much the game you create but the process you go through to create it. The objective is to create a new game. The first rule is that it has to involve physical activity."

"Can I just ask one question before we begin?" asked Kate.

"Sure," Doc said.

"Why are you guys really here? I mean why are you doing all of this with Annie?"

"That's two questions. But the simple answer to both of them is that Annie is here to lose weight."

"But I don't get it. She hasn't been to the Spa, Billy made her cry, she's shooting arrows, and she got whacked in the head with a Frisbee playing some game I don't even know the name of. Not to mention, we just tried fake pot! That's unlike any weight loss program I've ever heard of."

"Exactly. Shall we begin?"

"It's okay, Kate. Remember, you said to just go with it so let's just go with it. I trust, Doc," said Annie. "And it's nice to see him without his sunglasses." Annie smiled at Doc.

Doc dove in: "Okay, so remember the rules are that it has to be a new game or at least that you believe it to be a new game, involves physical activity, and each of you must contribute something to the creation of the game. I usually give groups about 10 minutes. Oh, and it should be a game you would like to play with your friends with a cool name. I'll be back in a few minutes. I forgot something at the house."

Doc didn't forget anything. He usually left the room during this activity so groups could feel total immersion in creating the game, no distractions, no opportunities to ask questions. Just figure it out on their own.

Kate and Annie were both lost in their thoughts, wondering how to get started. Both were still feeling a little buzzed from *Serenity Now*.

"Boy, am I glad we just took one little puff," said Kate.

"Me too," said Annie, thinking of Sam upstairs.

"Okay, what games do we like to play?" Kate mused. "Tennis... running..."

"Well, we used to like tennis and running," said Annie. "Can you like something even though you haven't done it in awhile?

"Sure. Take me with sex. I like sex but haven't had any in awhile," said Kate. They both laughed.

Annie flashed to her childhood. "I don't know why I thought of this but do you remember that one picture we looked at with us watching TV at your house in our PJs. Well, remember when our parents watched 'Laugh in' and we would all come over to your house and watch. Well, my favorite part of the show was 'Sock it to me'. This one woman—I forget her name—would always get tricked into saying that phrase and would get doused in water or something bad would happen to her. We would always start laughing just before she would get it. And she would just laugh it off. I used to think about that when I would get down in tennis and my opponent was just slamming me. I would say 'Sock it to me. I can take it.' And then it didn't seem so bad and I would start playing better."

"Why in the world would you think of that? What does that have to do with creating this game?" Kate asked.

"Nothing, probably," said Annie. "Must be the weed." They laughed some more. "Maybe we could create some kind of game where you just sock it to the other player, but they don't care," Annie said.

"You mean like dodgeball? Kate asked.

"Mmm, no, because there, you do care if you get hammered. It hurts." Annie said, as she rubbed her forehead.

"So you don't want it to hurt?" Kate asked.

"I guess."

Kate and Annie sat there mulling over their new game, or lack thereof. They were stuck.

Annie broke the silence: "Let's get back to tennis. We know we like tennis. What could we do with tennis that would make it different or new?"

"I don't get it. Why do we need a new game if we actually like playing tennis?" Kate frustratingly asked. "Why can't we just play tennis?"

"That's a good question, Kate. But if we liked it so much why haven't we played it in forever?" Annie paused, thinking. "I read something once about John Irving where he said all of his books were created by asking, What if...What if...What if—"

"What if we played without rackets?" Kate blurted out.

"What? You mean throwing the ball like a baseball instead of hitting it."

"Yeah, why not? Call it Tenbase."

"Cause we throw like girls."

"Yeah, that might not be much fun."

"What about something with doubles?" Annie asked. "You know, some kind of offshoot of the Australian Doubles we used to play with Sam, you know two against one."

"What would make doubles totally different? Something totally new?" Kate wondered aloud.

"I got it," Annie jumped up out of the sofa. "Are you ready?"

"What? What?"

"We play doubles but each side has only *one* racket," Annie said, holding up the index finger of each hand for emphasis. "Something you said earlier about no rackets just stuck in my brain. Maybe not no rackets, but what if each side had only one racket?"

"One racket?" asked Kate. "But what would the player without the racket do?

"Uh…Uh…we rotate. Take turns. That's it. We take turns. Call it *Turn Tennis,*" Annie said, as she twirled a 360.

"*Turn Tennis,*" I like it," said Kate. "Reminds me of my grandma saying, 'Now remember, Kate, wait your turn.'"

Kate jumped up and locked arms with Annie. They started jumping up and down, chanting "*Turn Tennis, Turn Tennis,*" turning with each jump, as giddy as school girls who just received a love note from a boy in the class. On one of the turns they both noticed Doc standing in the doorway, watching with amusement.

"DOC," shouted Annie. "We've got our game."

"I see," said Doc. "Something to do with bad dancing?"

Annie and Kate stopped.

"Well, sort of," said Annie. "We call it *Turn Tennis.* It's doubles with a twist."

"Sounds interesting."

"Hey, let's play it right now," said Kate, looking to Annie and then Doc.

"Yeah, why not," added Annie. "Do you play tennis, Doc?"

"Yeah. I'm a jack of all sports trades, master of none."

Kate slapped her forehead. "But can we get on the Spa tennis courts?"

"I'm not sure. It's almost midnight. I might be able to pull some strings."

"Pull them, Doc. Pull them," said Annie. "Kate and I will get changed and we'll meet you in five minutes on the path outside the shack…I mean Billy's house."

Both women dashed to get ready, Annie up the stairs, Kate to her room. Halfway up the stairs, Annie stopped suddenly and turned to Doc.

"Doc, we'll need another player. Can you find someone? Billy maybe? And we'll need tennis rackets. Do you have any?"

"I think so. But I think I only have two."

"Perfect."

Day 3
Play

Six

PLAYING THE GAME WITH NO NAME

As Doc hustled back to the shack, he knew he had some work to do. He wasn't used to people actually playing the games they came up with. Usually, when he did this exercise in class or in a corporate setting, he helped people process or debrief their experience in creating the game, helping them be more aware of how they might feel during the experience. Invariably, students or adults—didn't matter—would realize that when left free to create, they created something they would like to play with their friends. They felt energized, just like Kate and Annie. They could be themselves. The debrief discussion would then focus on how they could create a life that emulated *The Game With No Name*. From developing a game, most people recognized they had the power to do just that. But did they have the will, the courage to trust themselves?

How in the heck are we going to get on the courts? Doc wondered. Maybe we can climb over the fence. He pushed that problem out of his mind and made a quick call to address the other problem: the fourth player. One problem solved.

At the shack, he grabbed the two Jack Kramer specials from the sports bucket on the back deck. "We'll need a ball," he muttered to himself as he walked in the door off the deck. He spotted Obi, lying on the rug by the fireplace, eyes half shut, and realized there would always be a tennis ball near Obi. He patted Obi on the head as he grabbed the slobbery orb resting by his front paws. Best we can do on such short notice, he thought. Doc hurriedly changed and then rushed out to meet Kate and Annie who were walking over from their house.

"Hi, Doc." Annie whispered.

"Why are you whispering?" asked Doc.

"I don't know. It's late," as her voice returned to normal. "Did you see if Billy could play?"

"He wasn't around but I got someone else," Doc replied. "I was able to find the two rackets but I could only find one ball," as he tossed it to Kate.

"Oouuh, gross," said Kate. "It's all icky. What is this, the dog's ball?"

"Yep." Doc grinned.

"Are those wooden rackets?" Annie asked.

"Yep, Jack Kramer specials. Are you old enough to remember these?"

"Sure, my dad gave me one when I seven or eight," said Annie, as she took one of the rackets from Doc and rubbed her hand gently over the shaft. "Sweet."

"Well, we'd better get going," said Doc.

"Right," said Annie. "Do you think we can get on the courts?"

"I don't know," Doc replied. "Let's go see."

They walked quickly along the path lighted by the full moon. A few minutes later, as they neared the courts, Annie could make out the silhouette of a figure standing by the entrance to the courts.

As they got up close, Annie recognized her as the tennis woman.

"Hi, guys, Doc tells me you want to play some tennis. I'm always up for a game," she said, patting her tennis bag.

"Hello again," said Annie. "This is Kate, my friend."

"Chrissie," the woman said, shaking hands with Kate.

"Annie, why don't you explain to Chrissie the game you and Kate created. What are you calling it?"

"Oh…uh…well, are you sure we can get in?" asked Annie.

"Of course, I've got a key to the lock," said Chrissie, as she held up the key, which glistened in the moonlight. "Now tell me about this game," she said, as she slid the key in the lock.

"That sounds awesome," Chrissie said, after hearing Annie's explanation of *Turn Tennis*. "I'm up for it."

"What about lights?" asked Kate.

"Well, I'm afraid I don't have a key for those," said Chrissie. "Good thing it's a full moon tonight," she said, pointing to the sky.

They all looked up. It, indeed, was a full moon.

Annie thought about Sam's charge to have wild, full-moon sex with Billy.

"Beautiful," said Kate.

The catalyst in Doc came out and he took charge. "Okay, we only need two rackets. Do you want to use the Kramers or Chrissie's rackets?"

"We'd better use the Kramers," said Annie. "We're not really sure how this is going to go. But, hopefully, Chrissie has some better balls than the Obi ball."

Chrissie popped out a brand new can of Penns and everyone stopped so they could hear the air released upon opening. Anyone who has ever played tennis loves that sound.

"I think the teams should be me and Annie and Chrissie and Kate." Doc said. Doc enjoyed sizing up talent from years of making teams for faculty/staff pickup basketball games. Mentally he ranked, in order, Chrissie, himself, Annie, and Kate.

"Remember, only one racket per side and you have to take turns," Annie said, as players took their positions. "Other than that, I think we go by the regular rules of tennis.

Chrissie and Doc warmed up first. They then exchanged rackets with Kate and Annie, respectively, so they could warm up. Hitting with the wooden rackets felt strange.

"Should we practice taking turns or just begin," asked Kate.

"Let's just start," said Annie. "We'll figure it out as we go."

"Okay," Doc said. "Up or down."

"Down," said Kate.

Annie twirled the racket. "Up," declared Annie. "We'll serve. Here ya go, Doc," tossing him two of the balls.

As he prepared to serve, Doc noticed Chrissie and Kate discussing strategy.

"Hey, break it up you two."

Doc's first serve went into the net. His second serve was a little powder puff that Chrissie pummeled with her forehand for a winner before Doc was able to run over and hand the racket to Annie.

Doc's first serve from the Ad side was to Kate's backhand. As soon as he served he ran over to Kate and handed her the racket. Kate's return whizzed by before Annie could get her racket on it.

"Way to go, Kate," said Chrissie.

Doc and Annie looked at each other, realizing that they would need to be faster on the exchange.

"Love-thirty," Doc said as he prepared to serve, his eyes straining to acclimate to the moonlight. This time he served to Chrissie's backhand. He shortened his follow through and with a quick flick, tossed the racket as gently as he could to Annie. Annie, who had moved back away from the net, to give her more time to react, caught the racket with both hands and then quickly moved her hands to tennis grip. Chrissie's return, however, was headed toward Doc. Annie tried to move quickly but wasn't fast enough to cut the ball off. Love-forty.

"Good try, Annie," said Doc.

"Thanks for not hitting me in the head with the racket," she said.

"You're welcome."

Doc double faulted on his serve to Kate. First game to Chrissie and Kate.

"Should we change sides?" asked Chrissie.

"Sure," said Annie. "I think the moon was in Doc's eyes on that side."

"Hey, guys, I was watching you try to get to our returns," said Kate. "Pretty hilarious."

"Watch it, girlfriend, your turn is coming," said Annie.

"I have a suggestion," said Kate. "We should make a new rule that the ball has to be able to bounce twice in the court before going out. You still have to hit it on one bounce but this will force us to hit shots that the other team is likely to have more time to get to, you know, considering we have to pass the racket to our partner. And it adds a little more strategy as to whether you should hit the ball coming at you. If it's hard and long, it may bounce once and then out of the court before the second bounce, giving you the point. What do you think?"

After the threesome pondered that idea for a moment, Chrissie declared: "Brilliant, Kate. You show much promise as a Game With No Namer. I say we try it." Doc and Annie nodded.

As they switched sides, Annie took the deuce court. Doc decided to stand on the baseline and closer to Annie for an easier exchange of the racket. As Chrissie was about to serve, Kate was up near the T but she was facing Chrissie, her back to Annie.

"What are you doing?" asked Annie.

"You'll see," Kate responded without turning and giving a thumbs up to Chrissie.

Chrissie made sure her serve would be within the confines of the two-bounce rule, and upon completing the motion, immediately tossed the racket to Kate, who proceeded to drop it. Annie's return struck her square in the back.

"Sorry," said Annie. Fortunately, the ball hadn't been returned too hard.

Before the next serve to Doc, Kate and Chrissie tried a different strategy. Kate stood behind Chrissie on the baseline so that the racket could be exchanged more like a baton. When Chrissie served to Doc, Kate grabbed the head of the racket just as she finished her serving motion, and then moved around her into the court. Sensing that Kate was far back in the court, Doc hit a moderately risky drop shot that bounced near the other team's service line, which Kate could not reach.

"The Doctor, slicing them up," said Annie. "Good shot."

"Thanks," Doc said as he handed the racket back to Annie.

Chrissie's serve to Annie was good but wide and even though it was an Ace, it didn't make the two-bounce rule.

Love-forty.

Chrissie's serve to Doc hit right near the T. Doc lunged and got the racket out far enough to hit a weak return to the middle of the court. He quickly flipped the racket to Annie, who somehow caught it with her right hand on the shaft, as she moved near the net. After snatching the racket from Chrissie, Kate ran to her right to track down Doc's return and was able to hit a cross-court shot away from Doc. But Annie, quicker than Kate anticipated, was there in time to volley away the winner.

After a moment of disbelief, they all cheered, forgetting that it was well past midnight. They didn't care. Chrissie, Kate, Doc, and Annie had just played a fabulous point of *Turn Tennis*, a game that until a little bit ago did not exist. Annie relished in the moment as she turned to the baseline to begin her service game. Doc fist-pumped her: "Great shot, Annie."

"Nice toss, Doc," she said.

"Hey, Doc, I think I kinda get this," Annie said, just before serving.

"Good to hear. Welcome to *The Game With No Name*."

The players lost track of time, playing for at least two hours, experimenting at times with the most efficient ways to exchange the racket—sometimes they tried the toss, other times they tried the shadow method staying as close as possible to their partner for the quickest exchange. Annie and Doc got pretty good at tossing and catching. In one game, they had a contest to determine who could come up with the best throw and catch. Doc won with a behind-the-back flip that Annie was able to catch with one hand. The Jack Kramers got beaten up in that game with most of the throws crashing hard on to the court. If they were kids, parents watching would have told them to stop playing such a dumb game, "Someone's going to get hurt," they would have said. Every now and then,

Annie would shout "Sock it to me" just before Kate would serve, which made her laugh and disrupted her concentration.

The match ended with Annie spinning an Ace past Chrissie, who elected to let the ball go by, thinking that it would leave the court before the second bounce, but the ball nicked the baseline. Game, Set, Match to Doc and Annie.

After chatting with Chrissie for a few minutes, and thanking her for playing on such short notice, the three players walked back to the shack.

"Well, that was the most fun I've had in quite some time," said Kate.

"Yes, thanks, Doc, for setting it up," said Annie.

"Oh, I didn't do much," said Doc. "You guys came up with the game. That's a great *Game With No Name*. Good thing Chrissie had a key."

They walked the rest of the way in silence, basking in the feeling of exhaustion and exhilaration. Doc's natural inclination was to debrief, but he held back.

As they reached the shack, Doc said good night and reminded Annie of her body surfing experience with Billy in the morning at 8 o'clock. He placed the rackets back in the bucket and Obi's ball near his paws. Billy's light was out and Doc's was next in line.

Annie and Kate continued on towards their house. Annie looked for Billy in the swing, hoping he might be there, but it was empty.

Back at the house, the pot smell had dissipated. It looked like Sam had cleaned up a bit.

"Good night, Annie Oakley," said Kate. "Thanks for a fun night."

"Yea, too bad Sam missed it. I think she would have liked the game," said Annie, as she headed upstairs. "Good night, or should I say good morning."

As Annie walked up the stairs, she felt lighter, like something or someone was carrying her along. It was the most beautiful feel.

Seven

BODY SURFING WITH THE WHITE HORSES

As Billy waited for Annie, he walked along the shore, examining the nuances of waves as they rolled in—perfect for body surfing. He thought of his grandfather, who introduced Billy to life on and around the water. Not a day went by that Billy didn't miss him. Billy was probably eight or nine when his grandfather first told him his version of the White Horses.

"White Horse Island is a magical place, Billy," his grandfather stated one day while they hunted for shells after a high tide. "Do you know how this place became known as White Horse Island?"

"No, tell me, grampa," said Billy.

"Well, once upon a time, Poseidon, the God of the Sea, lived in a palace under the sea. He had an enormous stable filled with magical White Horses that pulled his chariot around all day and night so he could continually view his kingdom, which as you can see is vast."

"You mean he lived under the water?" Billy asked

"Yep."

"Cool."

"Poseidon was a mean God. He didn't treat his horses very well and made them pull his chariot around the underwater world, day after day after day, night after night after night. The horses worked all the time. They weren't allowed to play."

"They couldn't play?" asked Billy. "That would stink. I love to play."

"Do you want to know what the White Horses did?" his grandfather asked.

"What? What did they do?"

"Well, one day the leader of the White Horses began to plot the horses' escape. He was pretty sure the horses could get through the fence but he didn't know where they could go so that Poseidon couldn't catch them and bring them back. One of Poseidon's friendly dolphins, who was helping the white horse leader plan the escape, told him to go upward toward the surface of the sea and head for land.

"The magic of the waves will bring you to safety," said the dolphin. "Poseidon will never find you."

Finally on a night that Poseidon took a break from his chariot rides, the dolphin stole his trident while he slept and..."

"What's a trident," Billy asked.

"It's a big stick that has magical powers," his grandfather said. "Poseidon could do anything with it."

"Oh."

"The dolphin used the trident to open the fence's main gate and the horses, with their leader in front, fled the confines of the fence and headed to the surface. As they swam towards freedom, the sea rose up, the waves started their march. No one really knows why it happened. But using a full moon to guide them, the horses rode those waves all the way to the shore, to this very shore we are standing on right now."

"And where did they go?" asked Billy. "Where did the White Horses go, Grampa?"

"No one knows for sure," his grandfather said. "As they came to the shore, the moon dropped behind the horizon, just before the sun rose to the east. And in those few moments of darkness, all that was left were sets of human footprints in the sand leading away from the ocean right into the brush."

"You mean the horses turned into people." Billy said.

"Yes, people who loved to play and have fun because they never wanted to work another day in their lives. And Poseidon could never find them because he was still looking for horses."

"Wow," said Billy.

"You know, Billy, you might even be a descendant of the original White Horses. You love to play, don't you?" his grandfather asked.

"Sure, every day," Billy said.

"People will tell you that the story of the White Horses is just a legend, that it's not true. Don't you believe them. I've seen the White Horses with my own eyes."

"You have?" asked Billy, eyes wide with wonder.

"Yes, every now and then if you look closely, you can still see the White Horses playing in the water, as the waves dance to a perfect rhythm, curling up then folding over one after the other into the magical white foam."

"I see them," Billy said excitedly, as he pointed to the white caps."

"Me, too," his grandfather said. "Me too."

Annie waved as she saw Billy look up. Billy noticed that Annie was slouching less, a bit more bite in her step.

"Hi, sorry I'm a little late," said Annie. "We played this tennis game with Doc last night and didn't get home till two in the morning. I haven't done something like that in awhile."

"That's okay. I was just playing with the White Horses," Billy said.

"What?"

"Nothing. How was it?" asked Billy.

"Great," said Annie. "But I'm a little sluggish this morning." I'm not used to doing so much activity."

"Do you still want to try the body surfing?" Billy asked. "We don't have to do it now."

"No, no, I want to do it. I've only tried this a few times and I'm not really sure I was doing it right or not."

"Okay, the water's going to be a little cold when you first get in, so that will wake you up. But once you get moving around, you'll warm up.

"Okay."

Annie was scared to death. But she didn't tell Billy that. Scared of how she might react if he touched her, scared that she didn't really know how to body surf, scared that her weight would not let her do the things Billy wanted her to do. Scared of so many things. But something was drawing her to this moment.

"Basically, we're going to swim out to the sand bar, that's where the waves break," Billy said. "That's probably about 30 yards. You'll be able to touch bottom. I'll explain the rest when we get out there," Billy said, as he took off his shirt and placed it on one of the two chairs and towels he had situated near the water. "I assume you can swim."

"I'm very average," said Annie, as she took off her sun shirt to reveal her one-piece swimsuit, and oddly enough, did not feel embarrassed about her body in front of Billy.

"Good enough," said Billy. "Let's go."

Billy ran into the water and after a few yards dove in. Annie followed, a bit more tentatively. The cool water shocked her at first. They both stood up after the initial dive under the water.

"You don't need a spa to relax, refresh, or rejuvenate," said Billy. "Not when you've got this."

"I agree," said Annie. "This is awesome."

"Now, when we swim out, you can open your eyes underwater. It's not like there's chlorine in the ocean. The trick is to get your whole body and head into the water and relax. It's not a long swim."

"Okay."

As they began to swim, Annie exhaled slowly under the waves about 10 feet out and allowed her body to sink down towards the sandbar beneath her. She opened her eyes and looked around at the small fish that darted about. As she swung her arms through the water and kicked, she felt safe. Was it Billy making her feel this way or just good ole Mother Nature?

Annie popped up, breaking the surface, planting her feet on the sandbar. Billy was already standing.

"Good job," Billy said. "You're standing on a hardpack that is washed away and rebuilt every second of every day. That's how nature works."

"It was too short," said Annie. "I loved it."

"Well, let's see if you'll like body surfing," Billy said. "It's pretty simple, really. It's natural to be a little scared. Just think of yourself as part of the water. You're going to stand in front of me and I'm going to put my hands on your hips. You have to trust me. I'm just going to throw you into the waves. Put your hands out, tuck your head. Remember, you don't need to close your eyes. The water won't bother you."

Annie was listening closely, trying hard not be distracted as wave after wave crashed into her. She braced herself each time. Did Billy say he was going to put his hands on my hips? Stop acting like a schoolgirl, she told herself.

"The idea is to get right where the waves crest," Billy continued. "Once you feel it, you straighten out and your chest becomes the surfboard."

No wonder Billy was a very good bodysurfer, Annie thought. His chest was enormous, like a surfboard.

"Ready?" Billy asked.

"I think so," said Annie

Billy moved behind Annie as she bent slightly at the waist; she put her arms out and tucked. Billy put his hands on her hips and a few seconds later Annie was flying forward. As soon as she felt the wave she began flailing her arms through the water as fast as she could. Nothing. She stopped.

As she walked back towards Billy, he was laughing hysterically.

"What? What's so funny?"

"Nothing. Nothing. You looked like Doc in the water when he first tried this."

"I'm glad my performance amuses you," Annie said, laughing at herself. "What did I do wrong?"

"You tried too hard. You swam ahead of the wave. It couldn't catch up to you. You were all tense, instead of feeling the wave. You want to get right where the wave crests, about two thirds of the way up. Too far ahead or too on top, you'll just crash."

"Let's try again," Annie said.

She didn't flinch this time when Billy touched her hips. She inhaled and exhaled, timing the exhale with his toss. She tried to swim in a more relaxed fashion and felt the wave begin to carry her. I'm doing it, I'm doing it, she thought. A few seconds later—crash.

As she surfaced, she felt a little beat up. She didn't realize how forceful the water could be. She headed back towards Billy, turning and ducking each wave.

"So what happened there?" Annie asked as she neared Billy.

"Much better. You didn't stay straight and kind of veered into the face of the wave and it took you for a tumble. Again, feel the wave. Trust that the wave will take you for a ride.

"Yeah, I kinda got excited that I was doing it and that took me out of the moment," Annie said. "Let me just catch my breath a minute."

Looking to shore, Annie could see a couple of little kids right at the water's edge, digging in the sand.

"Okay, let's give this another try," said Annie.

Annie took a few deep breaths, relaxing the body, and again timed her exhale with Billy's toss. She began her relaxed stroke and felt the wave begin to carry her. She lifted her hips slightly and looked straight ahead, focusing on the little kids. What a feeling, being carried along by a force of nature. She rode a long way, until the wave and her swimming petered out. Annie stood up and rubbed the saltwater from her eyes and looked out to Billy. She couldn't believe how far she had traveled. Billy was clapping. She waved.

Annie turned back and couldn't believe how close she was to shore. She could see that the little kids had trucks and shovels. They never bothered to look up. Annie flashed to her own kids—Maggie and Dylan. Dylan was the one who worried her. He was so cute when he was little, just like those kids on shore. So athletic, so smart. Something happened in middle school. His growth spurt seemed to outpace his brain growth. He turned into somebody else, someone she didn't really know. That was around the time that John seemed to disengage as well. I need to call home today, she reminded herself.

Turning back to Billy she partly swam and walked back out.

"Nice job," said Billy.

"Thanks, I felt like I was really doing it," said Annie. "Let's try a few more.

Annie had some ups and downs on the next few tries but was enjoying both the rides and the crashes. Then, fatigue set in.

"I think this is it for me," Annie said, as she could feel her breathing becoming more labored. "I'm a little out of shape."

"You did outstanding for a first-timer," Billy said. "You're on your own for the last one," as Billy tucked and caught the next wave. Annie watched as Billy blended into the wave. It looked like he was using one arm as a rudder. He coasted all the way to shore.

Annie tried to visualize how Billy timed his tuck with the wave. She performed her breathing strategy. Relax, she told herself. She spotted the wave she wanted, tucked, and started paddling. Looking straight at Billy, she caught the feel of the wave and felt herself get lost in the wave. Before she knew it, she was looking at Billy's feet.

"Nice one," said Billy, as he helped her up.

"That was a blast," said Annie. "You looked like a dolphin on your run."

"Well, I pretty much start my day this way so I've learned a few tricks."

"You'll have to teach me," said Annie. "Oh my gosh, I just realized it's already Monday. I hope I don't run out of time. I'm leaving on Friday."

"Well, time is what you make it," said Billy as he tossed her a towel. "And by the way, you just burned about 400 calories."

"Now that's a fun way to burn calories," Annie replied. "Can we bring the ocean to Charlottesville?"

They both slumped into the chairs and looked out to Poseidon's sea.

Eight

LADDER OF SUCCESS

Annie had to admit that her physical attraction to Billy was getting stronger. She imagined her and Billy making love in the sand right here, right now. She tried to shove that image out of her mind.

Annie broke the silence: "I told Doc last night when we were playing our tennis game that I think I kinda get the whole thing. I mean I don't know why you guys are on my case, so to speak, but I felt different the moment I crossed that bridge to White Horse Island."

Billy was always leery when people would tell him that they "get it." He'd heard that many times from many people and then they'd go back to the world and act and behave as if they didn't get it.

"Well, my grandfather used to say that White Horse Island is a magical place," Billy said. "What do you get?"

"Well, that I have to do things that I like, try new things," Annie said, thinking of things she had tried over the past couple of days.

"Anything else?" Billy asked.

"Well, I'm still trying to figure some things out."

"It's pretty simple if you just trust the process."

"Really? Now that I don't get that," Annie said. "My life seems very complicated at the moment. It seems a mess, really. I don't make time for exercise. My eating habits are terrible. These last few days are the healthiest ones I've lived in awhile, well, if you don't count getting hit in the head by a Frisbee or smoking some artificial pot."

"I doubt your life is a mess. Why do you think that?" Billy asked.

"Do you really want to know?" asked Annie.

"What do you think?"

"Okay, I miss my daughter who just went off to college, my teenage son seems to be a train wreck waiting to happen, and my husband and I have gotten more distant. Add to that the fact that my job is pretty stressful, lots of pressure to perform, to make the bottom line at our Y—"

"I've heard this thousands of times," Billy interrupted, "not to dismiss your issues or anything, but everybody's got them, just different versions."

Silence.

"Are you going to make me cry again?" Annie asked.

"I am an asshole, as you've been told." Billy said.

Annie laughed.

"When is the last time you played with your son or husband?" Billy asked.

"What?"

"When is the last time you played with your son or husband? It's a simple question."

"I don't know. What does that have to do with anything?"

"If you don't know then it's been awhile, right?"

"Probably, but—"

"See those kids over there," Billy said, pointing over to the kids.

Annie looked a ways up the beach and saw the same kids she spotted while body surfing. A few more had joined them. Shovels, trucks, and buckets surrounded them.

"Yeah, sure."

"Go over and ask them what they're doing. Tonight, we will do whatever they tell you they're doing. But you can only ask them what they're doing. Nothing more."

"It's pretty obvious what they're doing."

"Go ask them."

"Okay, okay."

Annie got up and swiped the sand off her butt as she walked towards the kids. She felt awkward. She certainly did not want to spend the evening playing with trucks and building stuff in the sand…then again, she thought, what would be wrong with that, especially with Billy.

Surrounding a puddle of water were three boys and one girl. They were obviously making some kind of structure, maybe even a sand sculpture.

"Uh…hi guys," Annie said. "Whatchya doing?"

The little girl looked right at Annie, but didn't say anything. The smallest boy looked to be about four or five. The others were bigger, maybe a few years older.

"Playing," the smallest boy said without looking up. In fact, none of the other boys acknowledged her. Annie felt really stupid, but as she walked back to Billy she understood. Billy knew they were going to say that. She remembered when her kids were that age, that they answered the same question with the same answer. Whatever they were doing, they always simply said, "playing."

Billy had moved out of his chair and was lying on the sand, face down on his stomach, his chin resting in his crossed hands. He watched as Annie walked back shaking her head, smiling.

Annie lay down next to Billy, mimicking his position. Her body again came alive with sexual desire. This is getting ridiculous, she thought. They both watched the kids play for a few minutes, which helped Annie focus her attention away from Billy's body and back to their conversation.

"Okay, you got me," Annie finally said. "The kids said they were 'playing' as you knew they would."

"Now look at the parents and adults," said Billy, pointing.

As Annie looked in the direction of Billy's finger, she wondered why she hadn't noticed it before. There were no animals playing in the water, no dogs running around, very few pelicans flying. Even the sand crabs disappeared. And she understood why. Along the waterline, parents and adults sat in short, reclining beach chairs with cup holders, drinking and talking. Umbrellas hovered above them. Some had their earbuds—connected to their phones—planted firmly in their ears to take their minds somewhere else. They were definitely not playing.

"Okay, I get it," Annie said, trying hard not to look at Billy so she wouldn't get all flustered. "The kids are playing, the adults are not. I'm an adult. I have not been playing, not for myself and certainly not with my son and husband."

Billy let that sink in.

"How could I have let this happen?" Annie asked. "Is that why my life seems to be in such a mess because I don't play?"

"Again, I wouldn't say your life is a mess. It's just somewhat out of kilter. *When you play, you touch and feel that clean, unspoiled spot. It grows,*" Billy said.

"You mean like the stone with the walls around it that you showed me yesterday?" asked Annie.

"Yes, that stone is your spot. Touch and Feel are nature's way of introducing us to our world, but Play is nature's way of teaching us how to discover our gifts and turn them into skills."

"So that is what you guys have been doing with me, just playing," Annie said.

"More or less."

"But...but...that's so..."

"Simple? Yes, I know...but not easy."

Annie and Billy watched the kids playing, totally engrossed in shoveling, digging, and building.

"That makes sense," Annie said. "But why is it so hard?"

"Only you can answer that," said Billy, "but mostly because at some point you chose to climb the *Ladder of Success*. Here, let me show you." Billy walked over to the kids and talked with them for a few minutes. He came back carrying one of their plastic shovels.

"How did you get that away from them?" asked Annie, pointing to the shovel.

"I just told them that you were my wife and that you hadn't played in a long time," Billy said. "They just gave me the shovel without me even asking for it."

"So, now I'm your wife, am I?" teased Annie.

This time it was Billy's turn to blush. Billy started drawing lines in the sand with the handle-end of the shovel, which ended up looking like a ladder of sorts.

There were seven rungs to the ladder and Billy drew each rung so that they went a little outside the ladder on the right. He drew arrows on the top of each of the two sides of the Ladder, suggesting that the Ladder would keep going to infinity and beyond.

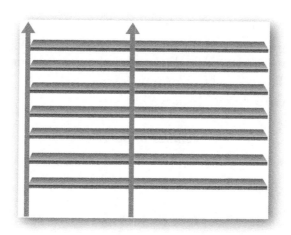

"Not bad," said Annie, "Did you major in art?

"No, English, but I've always loved to draw."

"Okay, so I see this is a ladder of some kind.

"Yes, it's the *Ladder of Success*," said Billy. "Most people start by striving to get good grades in school? Why?"

"Uh, so they can get into a good college?"

"Why?"

"So they can get a good job?"

"Why?"

"Okay, Okay, I get it."

Billy finished up the progression for her. "…So we can borrow money to buy a car…so we can get married…so we can borrow money to buy a house…so we can have kids…"

"…So we can help them get good grades in school…and so on…and so on," Annie said.

Billy drew some symbols on each of the lines.

"Well, that's quite a masterpiece, Rembrandt," said Annie. "How does this explain my predicament?"

"Well, like most people, you climbed this ladder, following a prescribed path. You started out with the best of intentions but somewhere along the way, you got lost because you didn't create a trail for yourself, and then you just did what was next. After awhile you were too high up to climb down, kind of like the cat stuck in the tree. You were afraid. And you thought that maybe, just maybe, if I climb high enough or long enough my life will feel—"

"Free, my life will feel free," Annie interrupted.

"But it doesn't, does it?" asked Billy.

Ladder of Success

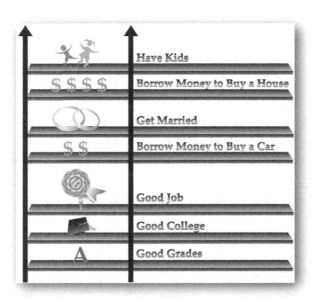

"No, I feel like a prisoner, like I'm a prisoner in my own body."

"That's what you have been feeling the past however many years. You've been feeling this yearning to find, to touch, to feel that clean unspoiled spot, that part that's right about you that you left behind as you climbed the Ladder."

"But I still like my job, I still love my family," Annie said, trying to defend her life of climbing. "Blah, blah, blah," said Billy. "Everyone says that or some version of that. It doesn't help how you feel inside—lost, lonely, with nowhere to go, no way out. You kept your end of the bargain, and it feels like a broken promise."

Annie let that sink in, not sure of what to ask or what to say.

"There is a way out, though," said Billy.

"How?"

"You've begun to experience it here at White Horse," said Billy. "Touch what's right about you. Feel what's right about you. When you do that, you begin to stop judging yourself and you stop inviting judgment from others, especially from your son and husband. You create your own trail."

"Why haven't I recognized this before?" asked Annie.

"When you are climbing up the rungs of success, your focus is on the next rung, not on how you want to feel. You can't choose what you don't know."

Annie saw the littlest boy who had been playing in the sand walking slowly towards them, looking a little timid, obviously ordered by the bigger boys to get their shovel back.

"Hi, sweetie," Annie said, trying to help the little boy be less afraid.

"Are you done playing with our shovel, ma'am?" the little boy shyly asked.

"We sure are," said Annie, smiling at the little boy, remembering the times she played with Dylan when he was the boy's age.

Billy handed the boy the shovel and he ran back to his friends, waving the shovel in the air like a trophy held high.

Annie turned away from Billy to hide the tears. Billy put his hand on her shoulder for comfort.

"I don't know why I keep crying," mumbled Annie. "I'm not usually like this." Billy knew not to say anything. The crying occurs when like and want collide.

Moments later, Annie turned to Billy, wiping away the tears. She wanted to kiss him, desperately; her lips touching his would make everything all right.

"We're going to have to stop meeting like this," Billy said, making Annie laugh and distracting her from her physical desire.

"That reminds me," said Annie, "I owe you a play date."

"A date? Now, Annie, you're a married woman."

"You know what I mean," said Annie, gently slapping Billy's arm. "But I think I've had enough of shovels and sand. "Why don't you and Doc come over to the house this evening and we can have a barbeque. I'd really like to have Kate and Sam get to talk to you guys some more. They don't really know what's going on. How about around six o'clock?"

"Sounds good, but I do the cooking," said Billy.

"Are you sure?"

"I'm sure," said Billy, as he dashed back into the ocean.

Annie started back to the house. When she neared the steps leading to the deck, she looked back and saw Billy lost in a wave. And the littlest boy was pouring water from a bucket on Billy's masterpiece, washing it all away.

Nine

HARRY'S EASY SPEED

*D*oc was on an errand run as part of the preparation for Billy's evening meal with Annie and her friends. Billy wrote everything down as to what Doc was to buy and where to go to do so—the SeaMarket, the Tomato Shack, the White Horse Wine Shop. Doc was pleased after Billy debriefed him about his body surfing experience with Annie. Annie seemed to be coming alive and paying attention to the spot, to what was right about her. They had kept her away from the dreaded Spa and, hopefully, Harry was keeping Sam occupied. Doc was still worried, however, that Annie would try to act on her physical attraction to Billy, which would ruin everything. Billy had to tell her what she was really going on.

Driving back to Billy's shack on Highway 12, Doc's thoughts floated to a conversation with Billy that helped solidify his view of how and why people move their bodies or eat what they do. Billy had started talking about energized information versus informed energy.

"When you feel what you do, when you hold on to what's right about you," Billy said, "you find energy sources to feed those experiences, to do the work that's necessary—informed energy."

At that moment, Doc realized that was the fatal flaw of most health and wellness programming experiences. The experts attempt to energize the information, to make the prescription more palatable. He began to see that most behavior change programs started with the behavior of interest, not the person of interest. Doc began to observe that most people attempting to follow the energizing information approach to health behavior change failed. They didn't move their bodies more or eat better because they were weighed down by their own lives. *They had to lose weight before they could lose weight.* Physical activity and eating nutritiously would then just become natural outcomes of living in a way that's aligned with one's *daimon*—personal destiny. When people discover this within themselves—and live it—they become weightless. They touch, feel, play, know, trust, and create their own feel of living.

Doc discovered this via his own autoimmune condition. The disease woke him up. He began stumbling upon and experimenting with anti-inflammatory diets. He observed that certain meals made him feel light, whereas some meals made him feel heavy. He paid attention to how food made him feel and started preparing more meals for his family with as much local produce as possible. He just started playing around with food.

Of course, Billy was way ahead of Doc. Billy knew for years that the way most people were living was weighing them down—that was the real energy crisis. That's why he left medicine, to explore feel. He didn't feel he could help his patients anymore, when most of them were weighed down by life. Through his interviews and his own experiences, he began to feel weightless, and he discovered food as a way to fuel his promise, the promise he had made to the White Horses years ago.

Doc's thoughts were interrupted when a Jeep passed him driving crazily fast on such a windy road. A man was driving with the passenger's blonde hair waving and glistening in the sun—Harry and Sam.

Annie and Kate had enjoyed their solitude the rest of the morning but after lunch began to wonder when Sam might return from her surfing lesson with Harry. Annie had filled Kate in on the body surfing and Kate was more convinced than ever that Annie was gaga over Billy. But Kate had to admit that Annie seemed happier than she had been in awhile. She wondered if it was Annie's silly crush on Billy or if Billy and Doc were actually making progress with Annie's case. She still found the whole "case" thing to be nonsensical. Who works on someone's case unbeknownst to that person? she wondered. How can you lose weight without going on a diet?

The quiet ended when Sam burst through the front door with Harry following close behind.

"Who wants to go play at the Y?" said Sam. "Harry wants to swim some laps and he said we can play in the Y's outdoor water park."

"Slow down, Sam. How was surfing?" asked Kate.

"Stupendous. Harry is a wonderful teacher," said Sam, as she wrapped her arm around his.

Kate and Sam couldn't believe how god-like Harry looked. He looked even better in the daylight. He had Sam imprisoned in some kind of trance as she didn't take her eyes off of him.

"Come to the Y with us," said Sam. "Harry said we can play around in the fun pool while he does laps."

Kate and Annie looked at each other, shrugged, and said "okay."

"Great," said Harry. "I'll introduce you to Bob." His voice still sounded like that of a Hollywood leading man.

"Yes, it will be fun to actually meet him in person," said Annie. "Give us a few minutes to get ready."

"You can just bring your suits and change there," said Harry. "Don't worry about towels."

As they were leaving, Doc pulled in the drive along side Harry's Jeep.

"Hey, Doc," said Harry.

"Going a little fast back there hey, Harry," said Doc.

"The need for speed, Doc, the need for speed," replied Harry.

"Wait, you two know each other," said Annie.

"Through Billy," said Doc. "Billy worked with Harry years ago and they became good friends."

"Worked on what?" asked Kate.

"Swimming," said Doc.

"Hey, Doc, why don't you come with us and tell 'em the story," said Harry. "Maybe it will help with Annie's case and all."

"Is there anyone in White Horse who isn't working on my case?" asked Annie.

"It appears not," said Sam. "but I certainly would be interested in hearing more about Harry's story, as she sidled up to touch Harry's body yet again."

Doc wasn't expecting Harry to reveal that he was in on the case and he was now worried that Sam would discover what was going on. He figured he'd better go along for the ride just to keep an eye on things and Harry's story might help Annie.

"Do you have enough room in the Jeep or should I drive?" asked Doc.

"We'll make room," said Harry.

"Let me drop off these groceries and I'll be right back," Doc said, as he grabbed the evening's meal and ran to the shack to unload. Before exiting the shack, he made sure to bring the DVD, the one that told Harry's story.

On his return, Doc squeezed in between Annie and Kate in the back. Harry zipped out onto Highway 12 to begin the 15-mile drive to the Outer Banks Y in Nags Head. Doc was glad he was in the middle because Harry's driving had them lurching from side to side the entire drive. Kate and Annie served as cushions as each of them hung on for dear life. Doc noticed that Sam had her hand on Harry's leg the entire drive, and the hand didn't budge even around the narrowest of turns.

Arriving at the Y, Annie was curious to see if Bob's Y was as service-oriented as her Y in Charlottesville. She prided herself on running a family-friendly facility. She had to admit, the Outer Banks Y was beautiful. Walking in, Harry was greeted with a warm "Harry, where have you been? We've missed you" from the woman working the front desk.

"Hi beautiful," Harry said in his exotic voice.

The woman blushed.

"I've got some guests with me, Dolores. They're going to play around in the outdoor water park while I do my laps".

"Sure, sure. No problem, Harry. You know you've got the run of the place."

"Is this guy a celebrity or something," Kate whispered to Annie.

"Is Bob around?" Harry asked.

"Oh, you just missed him. He just left to take a look at the new Y they're building. You know, the one up on Currituck Sound. Do you want me to reach him for you?"

"No, don't worry about it."

Harry waved and Dolores motioned them to enter with a big smile and wave of her hand. Annie registered a big check mark plus for Dolores.

"Have fun, ladies," said Harry, as he and Doc headed to the men's locker room.

"So what do you guys think of Harry?" asked Sam, as they changed in the locker room.

"Dreamy," said Kate.

"Exotic," said Annie. "He could be on TV."

"I've been having a blast with him," said Sam. "Hey, you guys don't mind that I'm spending time with him, do you?" she asked.

"Hey, you are single and free," said Annie.

"What about you and Billy?" asked Sam.

"Entirely different situation," said Annie, lying.

"Well, you know my feelings," said Sam. "We're here to have fun and he's a live one. Only a few days left."

"Let's go have some fun," said Kate, as she ran out of the locker room. "Bring your stuff so it doesn't get stolen."

They followed the signage to the outdoor pool. It was like a mini water park, complete with slides, volleyball net, and floating basketball hoop.

Annie was almost giddy. The pool was empty in the middle of the afternoon. They had the run of the place. They went down the windy slippery slides, played some volleyball, and shot hoops with a mini basketball. Then they spotted the water guns and sprayed each other, just like old times. Laughing, feeling free, before the onslaught of responsibility had caught up to them. They were playing.

I need to do this more frequently, Annie thought. What a great workout.

Kate was the one who spotted Doc. He was in a small room off the side of the pool. It appeared he was watching something on a TV.

"Let's go see what he's watching," said Kate.

"It's probably some porn," said Sam.

"SAM," said Annie and Kate.

They grabbed some towels from the pile, dried themselves a bit, and scooted into the room.

"Doc, what are you watching?" asked Annie.

"Do you want to see Harry Hopkins about 20 years ago?" Doc asked.

"I do, I do," said Sam, suddenly very interested in what Doc was watching.

Doc leaned forward. "Okay, it's quite a few years ago at the Olympics. Harry was the world record holder in the 100-meter backstroke and the heavy favorite going into the Games—"

"Wait a minute. Are you telling us that Harry Hopkins swam in the Olympics," said Annie.

"No way," said Kate. "I don't remember that."

"Way," said Doc. "Just listen to the story. Harry was prepared for his first Olympics to be the place where he would end his swimming career; he planned to leave the sport in glory. He was prepared to put it all out there, and then swim off into the sunset. As the games got closer, he began to listen to new voices. Voices that told him this would have to be the race of his life. Voices that told him no matter how much he had accomplished in swimming he was nothing until he won the gold medal. Harry began to listen to the voices. He began to believe that if he didn't win the gold all of his years in the sport were for nothing. So let's see how the race went."

Doc hit play as he had the race cued up.

"I see him," said Sam, "there he is, lane three. I'd know that beautiful bod anywhere. But he has no hair! Yuk."

They watched in silence as Harry made the turn in the lead. It looked like he would hold on. Five meters left to go and it looked like Harry would be taking home the gold. But the swimmer in the next lane was making up ground. At first, the American announcers thought Harry had won but then had to change their tune. The other swimmer had out touched Harry and beaten him by six one hundredths of a second. The camera showed the gold medal winner letting out primal screams while Harry, physically and mentally exhausted, laid his head on the lane divider.

Doc stopped the action.

"I had no idea Harry was an Olympic swimmer," said Sam. "He never said anything this morning."

"I could tell he was a swimmer," said Annie. "Look at those shoulders. But I don't know why I can't remember him. I'm sure I watched those games."

"So here's my question," said Doc. "Why do you think Harry lost?"

"Oh no," said Sam. "Is this one of your activities, Doc? This is for Annie's case, isn't it?"

"Sort of," said Doc. "So since you're Annie's friend and Harry's," looking directly at Sam, "just play along."

Sam nodded. "Stress," she said.

"Voices," said Annie.

"Thank you, students," said Doc, getting into prime professor mode. "Annie, what do you mean by voices?"

"Well, the voices of judgment and expectations," continued Annie. "The race became one of responsibility for Harry and he lost that freeness that you need to do anything well. He lost the playfulness because everyone else around him was so serious. He didn't protect his spot. He invited in the judgment. I know because it's happened to me. I've been hearing those voices for about fifteen to twenty years."

Kate and Sam's jaws dropped. They had never heard this kind of language from Annie. It was like she was speaking in a foreign tongue, like she was Harry Potter.

"Go sister," said Kate.

"Wow, Annie, I leave you for one morning," said Sam.

"Well, you missed the tennis thing too," said Annie. "You were stoned, remember?"

"What tennis thing?" asked Sam.

"We'll tell you later," said Kate.

"So what do you think Harry did after the Olympics?" asked Doc.

"Opened his surf shop?" asked Sam.

"Nope," said Annie. "I bet he found Billy Pelican."

"Right again, Annie," said Doc. Doc went on tell them how Harry met Billy and how it couldn't have been more perfect timing for both of them. Billy was beginning his quest to find a life outside of medicine and Harry was a mess. They sat down together and started to talk. Harry shared his life's story with Billy and began to describe what he called *Easy Speed*, which he considered to be a feeling of harmony with the water. He was at his best when he felt he was swimming to 100% of his ability with only 80% effort. He felt so engaged in what he was doing that he was gaining energy while doing it. Harry knew that this was how he felt after a race he won, after a race that he did great in. Billy suggested that Harry create his life around *Easy Speed*, but, at first, Harry resisted. He didn't believe that *Easy Speed* was something he could create. Harry believed it was something that happened by accident. Fortunately, Billy won the argument. The reality was that Harry could train for *Easy Speed*. He could train to feel the way he wanted to feel in the water. He would have to practice by preparing. He engaged in the feel he liked to have and learned how to create it. It took him more than three years to quiet the voices. And then four years later it was time for the next Olympics.

"So what happened?" asked Kate. "I can't believe I don't remember Harry Hopkins. I guess I was more of a track and field fan."

"Well, let's see," said Doc, who had the race cued up and ready to go.

The announcers were highlighting Harry before the race and wondering aloud if he could finally win Olympic gold.

"There he is," said Sam. "Lane four. Still no hair."

As the race unfolded, Harry began to pull away from the field. With five meters to go it was obvious that Harry was going to win. As he touched the wall, the announcer said, "Hopkins finally wins Olympic gold."

The three women cheered.

The camera showed Harry, his right arm raised high, looking to the stands, smiling. His mother was crying, hands over her mouth. No matter how many times Doc showed and viewed this clip, he had to fight back tears. He knew Harry's mom had died from cancer a few years later. He couldn't bring himself to tell the three women.

In a post-meet interview, Harry said he won because for the first time in his life he brought himself to the race, what was right about him. "I just reminded myself that I was at practice, playing in the water," Harry said. "And then the race was over."

Doc stopped the DVD.

Annie began to cry. She didn't care anymore about holding it in.

"What's the matter, honey," said Kate, as she put her arm around Annie.

"I…want…to…bring…myself…to…the…race," Annie said, in between the tears and sobs.

"What?" asked Sam.

"I want to bring myself to the race," Annie repeated, this time with more conviction.

Doc spotted a box of tissues in the corner of the room and brought them over to Annie.

"Do you have to make her cry *all* the time?" asked Sam, looking directly at Doc.

Doc shrugged.

"It's okay, Sam. Doc knows what he's doing. I'm okay. It's just my spot. It's growing. Since I've been here, my spot's been touched. I can feel it. I feel alive. I feel more like myself than ever before."

On cue, Harry walked in.

"My hero," said Sam, as she jumped into Harry's unexpecting arms.

The women were relatively quiet in the locker room as they toweled off and changed back into their street clothes. Sam was happy as she was anticipating having sex with an Olympic gold medalist. Kate was happy because her friend was discovering herself. Annie wasn't quite sure how to feel.

Harry and Doc were waiting in the lobby as the women walked out. Annie trailed, mulling over her experiences. As she walked by the desk, Dolores waved her over and whispered, "Good luck with your case, honey."

Ten

TUMBLING DOWN THE DUNES

*H*arry was born and raised in Nags Head. He learned to swim in the ocean and later honed his skills at the very Y he and his new fan club had just left. After the first Olympics fiasco, Harry was so distraught he had contemplated suicide. Billy saved him and he would do anything for Billy. Once Billy filled him in on Annie's case, he was more than happy to keep Sam occupied. The problem was he was beginning to like Sam. Her body had looked incredible on the surfboard. She was shallow but, being honest with himself, so was he. Maybe something could come from this, he thought.

On orders from Billy, Harry was to keep everyone occupied a little longer in the afternoon—so Billy could begin meal preparation at Annie's house with no distractions. Harry knew just where to go, and it was only a few minutes drive from the Y.

"Are you guys ready for another fun workout?" Harry asked, as he pulled into the park's parking lot a few minutes later.

"What time is it?" asked Annie.

"It's about four," said Doc, who, being a Type A, always knew what time it was.

"Well, as long as we're back by six or so," said Annie. "Billy's coming over to cook us dinner," saying it as an announcement so everyone could hear. Doc and Harry, you're invited too." Of course, Doc already knew.

"Ohhhh, dinner with Billy," teased Sam. "Can you make it, Harry, please?"

"I'm sorry, I have plans this evening," he said. "But Billy is a great cook. You'll enjoy it." This news didn't erase Sam's pouty face. "And, Annie, this won't take long. We'll be back in time." A few minutes later Harry pulled into a parking lot.

"What is this place?" asked Kate.

"It's Jockey's Ridge State Park," said Harry.

"It doesn't look like much," said Sam, still pouting.

"You'll see," said Harry.

They followed Harry down the boardwalk through the trees and when they came out the other side, they were surrounded by sand and sand dunes as far as the eye could see.

"Meet the tallest dunes in the United States," said Harry.

"Wow," said Annie, as she looked out to see sand rising up in various places.

A short walk later they were at the bottom of the highest dune, about 100 feet. People were rolling down, running down, and boarding down the steep dune, laughing while doing it.

"Okay, shoes and socks off. We're going up," said Harry. "Years ago I used to run up these dunes for training."

"I'll wait here for you guys," said Doc. "I get a little vertigo with heights."

"Oh, c'mon, Doc, it's not like it's Mount Everest," said Kate, who had already flipped her socks and shoes off. "I'll hold you at the top so you don't fall off."

"Yeah, c'mon, Doc. We're not going up without you," said Annie.

Doc begrudgingly took his shoes and socks off and placed them in the pile.

Sam grabbed Harry's hand for some help about halfway up. Doc took the lead and Annie noticed from the back that Doc was a little bowlegged but had very athletic legs—runner's legs. Annie and Kate brought up the rear. Annie's legs were feeling the tennis and the bodysurfing. She felt heavy.

Doc slowed to let them catch up and they all reached the top at about the same time. The view alone was worth the trip.

The Roanoke Sound was to the east with the ocean to the west. It seemed as if sand, water, and sky all merged together to form a magical gift of nature.

Off in the distance, Annie saw hang gliders and kites flying.

Doc sat down to help him stay balanced. Kate plopped down next to him to keep him company. Harry and Sam did the same.

"Well, what do you think?" asked Harry.

"It's incredible," said Annie, still standing and taking it all in.

"Yeah, it's my favorite place," said Harry.

After a few minutes of silent wonder, including even Sam, Harry rose up like a camel preparing to trek across the Sahara. "It's time to go," he said as he fell to the sand, tucked his arms to his chest, and began his roll to the bottom.

"HARRY, WAIT FOR ME," Sam cried out, as she began her roll to catch up.

"Okay, Doc, are you ready?" asked Kate.

"I think I'll walk down," said Doc.

"C'mon you slow pokes," said Annie as she moved into roll position and took off.

"Oh no you're not," said Kate to Doc, as she darted behind him and gave Doc a solid push in the back. Doc tried to grab his sunglasses. Too late. They flew off as he began his head over heels tumble to the bottom. He was out of control and going too fast to stop. He made sure to close his eyes to protect them.

As Doc neared bottom, he somehow got his feet underneath him and was able to get into an upright position, resembling an ape to man transformation. He ran the few remaining feet to flat land and then stumbled around like a man who had too much poof juice before falling flat on his back.

"Doc, are you okay?" asked Kate. "I'm so sorry. I didn't mean to push you that hard." Doc raised both arms and flashed both middle fingers, which was becoming his signature move these days.

"Okay, he's good," said Harry, as he and Annie grabbed his arms and pulled him to his feet. Doc was still a little woozy as he tried to spit out the sand from his mouth.

"My thunglathes. Did anyone get my thunglathes?" he asked. His mouth was bone dry, the heat and his autoimmune condition were not a good combination.

"I've got them, Doc," said Kate, who could not contain herself any longer and just burst out laughing as she handed the glasses to him. Then, Harry, Sam, and Annie joined in. Doc looked like he had just tumbled around in a dryer. Doc could only smile.

"Thith ith definithly not my favorith path," said Doc, as he grabbed his shoes and socks and headed for the Jeep with the rest of the gang having a rollicking good laugh behind him.

Eleven

Sam's Naked Body and the Arrow

*I*n 1975, the summer that Billy turned 14, Billy's father and grandfather had a falling out and his father took a government job in DC. Billy was crushed. He loved the Outer Banks, the ocean, and his grandfather. He begged to stay but his father said moving to DC would be the best thing for him. Billy could visit his grandfather during the summers.

Near the end of summer, the night before they were to move to DC, Billy's grandfather drove Billy to the shack property and told him of his plans to build a beach house for him.

"But why here?" Billy asked. "So far from your home."

"Because, remember, Billy, this is where the White Horses play," his grandfather said. "You'll be able to call to them right from the back deck."

"I don't want to move to DC, grandpa," Billy said, tears welling up.

His grandfather put his arm around Billy. "Oh, you'll be fine, Billy. You're smart as a whip and a great athlete. You'll easily make lots of new friends."

"But I'll miss you," Billy sniffled.

"I'll tell you what. Every time you miss me, just call up the White Horses in your mind's eye. They have magical powers and will come get me to take me right to you. It will be like I'm right there playing with you—me and the White Horses."

Billy nodded.

"And, remember, the White Horses are always here waiting to play with you when you return."

*B*illy Pelican was fast at work inside Annie's rental house. Cooking came as naturally to him as playing basketball. And once he left medicine, he had even more time to perfect the fine art of preparing foods with locally grown produce. He wasn't a master chef, not anything near that, but the food he prepared always had a healthier taste to it; you felt lighter after eating Billy's meals and his cooking was the one thing all of his ex-girlfriends raved about. They wanted him to love them as much as he loved cooking for them, but it never happened. Billy was a life detective; there wasn't much room in his life for anything else.

Billy wanted dinner close to ready when everyone arrived so he could spend some time with Annie. As he fired up the grill on the back deck, Billy wondered why Annie hadn't yet asked why he had selected her for his first official White Horse Island case. He wasn't sure what he would tell her, since she had really chosen him.

Billy's thoughts were interrupted by the front door slam and the sound of voices.

"I'm taking all of my clothes off right here to get all of this sand out. It's everywhere."

"Sam, don't do that. That's not decent," said Annie. "I don't need to see your naked body,"

"Whose body do you want to see, Billy's?"

"No."

"Oh, yes you do."

"Sam, don't."

Sam began running through the house, flipping her clothes off as Kate and Annie tried to catch her, laughing. She made it to the kitchen and that's when she noticed Billy giving the thumbs up sign from the deck. Billy had seen many women's naked bodies, and for forty-eight, Sam had a good one.

"AAHHH," screamed Sam. "What the fuck is he doing here?" pointing at the window. She backtracked her way out and made it to her room, slamming the door behind her.

Annie and Kate spotted Billy on the deck and he motioned for them to come out.

"Billy, what are you doing here?" asked Annie. "You scared Sam half out of her mind. And you saw her naked, Ouhh."

"Sorry about that," Billy said, smiling. "But somebody probably needs to scare her a bit anyway."

"Hey, she's our friend," said Annie.

"Is she?" Billy asked, still smiling.

"Yes, she is. Why are you smiling?" Kate asked.

"Because it was funny." Billy said.

The women couldn't help themselves. They started laughing. And could not stop. Finally, Annie slowed down long enough to remember her original question: "But what are you doing here?"

"I'm making you guys dinner like I said I would," Billy said. "I hope you don't mind that I let myself in."

"Well...uh..."

"Where's Doc?" asked Billy, quickly changing the topic.

"He was going to take a quick dip in the ocean to get all the sand out," said Kate. "We were full of sand from Jockey's Ridge. You should have seen Doc."

Both Kate and Annie started laughing again as they both visualized Doc tumbling down the sand dune. Annie laughed so hard her stomach started hurting.

"Sorry, I missed it," said Billy. "Why don't you guys get showers and I'll finish up dinner."

"What are we having?" asked Annie, as she tried to catch her breath.

"It's a surprise."

"Party pooper," said Annie, as she and Kate left to try to get Jockey's Ridge sand out of the crack of their butts.

*D*oc saw Billy on the deck and climbed the windy, weather beaten steps to reach him.

"So how'd it go?" asked Billy.

"Pretty good, I think," replied Doc. "After *Easy Speed*, she said she felt it, that she felt like herself for the very first time. She also mentioned something about judgment or being judged."

"Good. Oh, I should warn you that a few minutes ago I saw Sam naked. She freaked."

"Well, you do attract women like bugs to a windshield. I won't even ask how that happened."

"Yeah, well, let's get back to work. Set the table. Open the wine. Make yourself useful. Annie's getting close to the like versus want distinction."

Billy knew that the hard work was to come for Annie. She would be tested. The Touch, the Feel, the Play were the starting points, the entryway to the feel of one's life. Annie had to feel the difference between wanting something and liking something. Liking led to creating one's own path, and, ultimately, weightlessness. But to experience that you had to get off the path that everyone else was on, and by which they judged you, if you let them. You couldn't choose what you liked if you didn't know it, if you stayed on the path of judgment by climbing the endless Ladder of Success.

"*B*illy, I can't get Sam to come out of her room," said Annie. "She says she's too embarrassed."

"Hard to believe," Billy said. "It's nothing I haven't seen before."

"Billy!" said Annie.

"Okay, Okay, I'll try to get her out," said Billy. "Start in on the appetizers and the salad."

Annie, Kate, and Doc were famished. They hadn't eaten much during the course of the day. Doc offered the women some wine and they started in on the salad and crab cakes.

"I couldn't get her out," Billy proclaimed, as he returned a few minutes later.

The food was intoxicating as was the wine.

"SAM, C'MON," shouted Annie. "THE FOOD IS SOOO GOOD."

"What day is it," said Kate. "I can't even remember how long we've been here."

"It's Monday evening," said Doc.

"Already, wow, I've been having so much fun," said Kate.

"Me too," said Annie, as she grabbed another crab cake.

"Ready for entrees?" Billy asked as he brought in the foil wraps and placed them in front of Doc, Kate, and Annie.

The grilled salmon with homemade basil pesto sauce and tomatoes was scrumptious, so good they all forgot about Sam. Both Billy and Doc had their own thoughts about how to proceed following dinner, but the doorbell interrupted their next move.

Sam dashed out of her room thinking it might be Harry and opened the door only to see a FedEx guy with a package in hand. "Package, are you Annie Jackson?"

"Uh…no…but she's staying here," said Sam, clearly disappointed.

Doc and Billy looked at each other, wondering if either of them had set this up. They both shrugged.

Doc took advantage of the moment. "Wait a second," he said, while grabbing Annie by the arm to guide her to the door to get her package. "C'mon, Kate, you too."

"I wasn't expecting a package," said Annie as the FedEx guy handed her the envelope. "Hey, Doc, is this part of the case?" asked Annie. "Do you know, Doc?" directing her question at the FedEx guy.

"No, Ma'am, I just deliver packages," he replied.

"Excuse me, but would you mind if we took a look at your truck for a minute?" asked Doc.

"Well, I'm in a bit of a rush," said the FedEx guy.

"It will only take a minute," Doc said. "C'mon, Annie and Kate. You can come too if you want, Sam."

"Sam can stay here," Billy said, who had made it to the door. "I'll catch her up on dinner," trying to introduce a truce.

Sam, who hadn't eaten since she had lunch with Harry, reluctantly agreed, and closed the door after them. She was now alone with a man who had seen her naked without having sex with her—a rarity. Of course, both Billy and Sam had seen their fair share of naked women and men. Under different circumstances they might have been rolling in the sack together.

Outside, Doc was looking at the side of the truck, where the large "FedEx" logo was placed.

"Look at the logo, said Doc. "What do you see?" he asked.

Annie and Kate looked hard. All they saw were the purple and orange letters. Nothing else.

"Why don't you move back a bit," said the FedEx guy, who was on to what Doc was having them look for. "Sometimes that helps."

As the women moved back, Kate saw it first. "Hey, I think I see an arrow," she said.

"Where, I don't see anything," said Annie.

"Here, right, here," said Kate, as she walked up to the truck and outlined the arrow with her finger between the E and the X.

"Wow," said Annie. "I've never seen that before."

"Yeah, that's our arrow," said the FedEx guy. "It guides us to our next destination. We're always on target. Stuff like that."

"Cool," said Annie, as she thought of shooting arrows with Ian and Mac. "I just can't believe I've never seen it before."

"Me either," said Kate.

"Well, now that you've seen it, you can't not see it," said the FedEx guy. "Have fun with your package," as he hopped in the truck and drove around the cul-de-sac, waving as he drove to his next destination.

"You wanted me to see the arrow, right, Doc," said Annie. "Why?"

"Well, it's cool mostly," said Doc.

"I haven't known you long, Doc, but there's more to it," said Annie.

"Well, I like metaphors, and I like the arrow as the metaphor for the spot…"

"I knew it," interrupted Annie. "The arrow is like our clean, unspoiled spot. It's subtle, so it has to be touched, to be felt, or you will miss it, or, you know, cover it up. But it's always there no matter what."

"Excellent," said Kate. "I like it."

"And how do you do that?" asked Doc, ever the professor.

"PLAY," shouted Kate and Annie together.

"And what have you been doing since you've come to White Horse Island?" asked Doc.

"PLAYING," they shouted in unison. Annie and Kate fist-pumped each other.

Doc couldn't help but smile at their enthusiasm.

"And some of that play has been directed by you, Annie." Doc reminded her. "Play is a natural process that draws out your personal expression."

"Okay, I'm starting to get it," said Kate. "But how does all this help Annie lose weight? That's what I don't get. I mean at some point doesn't she need to follow a diet of some kind."

"I got this one, Doc," said Annie. "The way I get it, Kate, is that since Billy and Doc have been on my case, I have felt more alive, more myself, and to be honest, in some ways for the very first time."

"Informed energy," interjected Doc, "rather than trying to energize information, which is what most programs do, whether it be weight loss or diets or whatever."

"Right," continued Annie. "And they all make me conform to something I'm not. I have to give up a piece of myself to comply with the program, which is exactly what you don't want to do."

"Right," said Doc. "That's why the data show that in the long term the people who are positively impacted by these programs are the experts who develop and offer them."

"But aren't you guys kind of experts?" asked Kate.

"I suppose, but we'd like to think that we are experts in helping you find and interpret the clues to be your own expert. Billy is the best at that. I'm learning.

Kate and Annie mulled this over.

"Here's the thing," continued Doc, "you don't need experts and all of their prescriptions, techniques, and diets. There's a great book called *Defining the Wind*, about this guy who went on a journey to discover the essence of wind and how it's measured. At the end of his investigation, he simply concluded that '*our body* is the greatest perceptive instrument ever designed. Not only can it perceive sound, light, aroma, taste, and time, it has the ability to process, organize, and categorize massive amounts of data and to find the utility, value, and meaning in that data.'"

"I never thought of my body in that way," said Annie.

"And I'll go further," said Doc, who was on a roll. "The experts come along and make you question this ability of your own body. And if you haven't been paying attention to the magic that your own body possesses, you judge yourself as insufficient and give yourself up to these experts, thinking that they must have the weight loss answers for you."

"But they don't," said Annie. "They can't."

"Okay, so Annie is discovering her body, her self," said Kate. "She's the expert. I get that. But that seems kind of easy to do when she's on vacation. How does she do that in the real world, you know, when she gets back?"

"Well, I don't agree completely there with the easy part," said Doc. "Look at how many people go on vacation and then come home saying they need a vacation to recover from their vacation. But I think answering your question, Kate, is going to take some more wine," said Doc. "We'd better get back inside and see how Billy and Sam are getting along."

While Doc was outside with Annie and Kate, Billy played nice and served Sam the crab cakes, salad, salmon, and wine. He cleaned up while Sam ate.

"Do you want some more wine?" asked Billy.

"Sure," said Sam.

When Billy came over to refill her glass, Sam grabbed his left wrist, the one without the wine and said in a calm voice: "I know you don't like me, and the feeling is mutual, but Annie is my friend, and I think she wants to have sex with you. I think it would be the best thing for her."

Billy stayed calm and finished pouring the wine as Sam let go of his wrist. Billy sat down next to Sam and looked her in the eyes.

"I don't think you're a very good friend to Annie at all," said Billy with such steely resolve that it filled Sam with fear. "I don't think you know her at all. You think she should have sex with me because that's all you know. That's what you want to do."

"You son-of-a-bitch," said Sam, standing up. "You don't know anything about what I want."

"Yes, I do," said Billy, who stood up as well. "I bet after I saw you naked, you ran into your room and thought about having sex with me because that's all you know."

Sam slapped Billy across the face. Then she kissed him, hard. Billy pulled away.

"I guess I know you better than you thought," said Billy. "Just stay out of the way so Annie can lose weight. And don't you hurt, Harry. He and me are real friends."

"I'll do whatever I want with Harry. He likes me."

"You wouldn't know what *like* is if it came up and bit you in that tight little ass of yours."

"See, you know you want me and my ass," said Sam, who turned her back to Billy and bent over so he could get the full effect, just as Doc opened the door.

Sam quickly stood up. "Everything all right?" asked Doc, who hesitated a bit so that the tension could diminish before Kate and Annie walked in.

"Sure, fine," said Sam. "Billy and I were just discussing…uh…our love lives."

"Oh, I bet that was interesting," said Annie, as she and Kate followed Doc inside. "You two getting along?"

The wine was getting to Sam. "Famously," Sam replied. "We both think that you should just have sex with him and get it over with."

And with that, Sam walked to her room and slammed the door behind her.

"What…what…what did you do to her, Billy?" demanded Annie, who was embarrassed to the tilt.

"I didn't do anything," said Billy. "Sam is just confused about the difference between having sex and making love. And I didn't agree with her when she said we should have sex."

"Well, I think you'd better leave," Annie said, who didn't know how else to handle the situation. She wanted to run and hide.

Billy knew better than to argue his case and walked out the front door. Doc followed him out.

"You've got quite the effect on women," said Doc as they made the short walk to the shack. Billy said nothing. "What do we do now?" asked Doc.

"We wait," said Billy. "We wait for Annie to come to us."

"Good," said Doc, "because I've still got sand in my butt to get out."

Twelve

WILD HORSES AND THE SWING

After Billy and Doc left, Annie and Kate both agreed that it was best to just lay low that night and regroup in the morning. The explosiveness between Billy and Sam had put a damper on what had been an otherwise fun-filled day.

Annie took her FedEx package and moved out to the deck. The sound of the waves and fading light relaxed her. Inside the envelope was a DVD with the words "Annie@WHI" written on the disc. No name, no return address, no idea who it was from. She put the DVD back in the envelope, reminding herself to view it later.

Annie closed her eyes and reviewed the day's events, which began with *Turn Tennis* and body surfing and ended with water play at the Y, Jockey's Ridge, and a great dinner. She felt like she had soaked up the day's events. She honestly felt lighter, her body more alive. Something Billy said got her attention: having sex versus making love. Why was she so attracted to Billy? Was it about sex or love? She laughed to herself. *I don't even know what love is.* She seemed like such a contradiction: she felt more like herself than ever before after just a few days with two strangers than in all of her years with John and the kids, the people she was supposed to love. *How can that be?* She was afraid of going back and falling into the same pattern. Maybe she had just forgotten the special moments, a prisoner of the present. Was it her fault that things had turned out the way they had? Everyone just doing their own thing. It bothered her that she didn't play with John or Dylan, yet playing with Billy and Doc was so easy, so natural. No judgment. Maybe I do invite judgment from John and Dylan. Why would I do that? How did Billy know to ask me that question?

Annie's cell phone rang. It was Dylan.

"Hi honey," answered Annie.

"Hi mom."

"Whatchya doing?" Annie asked, envisioning the little boy from the beach this morning who reminded her of Dylan.

"Dad and me are finishing up pizza. I went to open gym tonight."

"That's great, Dylan. How did you do?"

"Well, not too good. I ain't that good compared to the other guys but I made a couple of shots."

Annie hated Dylan's grammar but she didn't correct. "Well, remember, you're only a freshman, and you haven't played much. How was school?"

"Okay, I guess. In history, we learned about pirates. Did you know that Blackbeard hid out on the Outer Banks, probably right where you're staying.

"I didn't know that," said Annie.

"Our teacher told us a pirate joke. Want to hear it?"

"Sure."

"Where do one-legged pirates love to eat breakfast?"

"I have no idea."

"IHOP. Get it mom. I…HOP."

Annie laughed out loud. "Good one, Dylan. You must be a one-legged pirate because that's your favorite place to eat." Annie envisioned Dylan scarfing down pancakes.

"Well, I gotta take a shower and do my homework. Dad says he'll talk with you tomorrow. He's got to clean up and get some work done."

"Okay, honey, love ya. Thanks for calling."

"Bye, mom."

One of our better conversations, Annie thought. At least he was interested in something. Hopefully, this year would be better than the middle school hell they lived through last year. Of course, John didn't want to talk but he probably was tired. Annie's body, although tired, was urging her to move it. This surprised her. She scooted down the deck stairs to the path out back—the path to the Spa, the path that everyone walked on.

Annie remembered Billy's question that first day, "Do you always walk on the path?" Moments of her life flashed—winning states, graduation day, meeting John at UVa, marriage day, the births of Maggie and Dylan, being named executive director for the Y. She was living the Ladder. She thought, I did what I was supposed to, it doesn't feel how I thought it would, I don't know what to do about it. But I do know what to do about it—touch, feel, play. Annie kicked off her flip flops and let them lay where they fell.

She walked off the path and on to the beach.

The sand felt heavenly, so soft and forgiving. She headed towards the sound of the waves. It was like she was walking on air. She never felt so light. As she reached the water's edge, the crests of the waves appeared to her as White Horses. They were dancing, playing, whispering to her to come join them, to wonder, to dream, to be childlike. Am I dreaming? she wondered. And then they were gone.

A thunderous sound from up the beach woke Annie from her dream-like state. She turned to see the wild horses galloping towards her, the white horse in the lead. Instead of running to the side out of the way, Annie panicked and began to run down the beach in the direction the herd was going. The stampeding herd was quickly gaining on her. Fear made her try to run faster, to no avail. In a moment she would be trampled, a tragic vacation story.

A massive figure came out of the dark of the ocean, picked her up like she was a toothpick, and carried her to safety, driving them both into the sand as the horses roared by where Annie had just stood.

Annie couldn't breath. It took her a few seconds to realize that she was alive, covered in sand, but alive. As she recovered, her breathing started.

She coughed sand out of her mouth. She was able to sit up, swipe the hair out of her eyes, and open.

Billy, beautiful Billy Pelican. But how?

"Are you okay?" Billy asked.

"I…think…so," said Annie. "How…how did you do that? Where did you come from?"

"Well, I was running back from the pier and I heard the horses, then I spotted you. Good thing you had a white shirt on. What were you trying to do, outrun the horses?"

"I…I…I panicked. I don't know what I was doing," said Annie.

"C'mon let's get you some water at the shack," said Billy, as he helped Annie get to her feet.

"I…I…I don't know if I should," said Annie, not trusting herself alone with Billy.

"It's all right, Annie. You can just sit on the swing and I'll bring it out to you. Okay?"

"Okay."

They walked in silence to Billy's shack with Billy's arm around Annie's shoulder, her body alive with excitement. Billy headed inside and Annie walked over to the swing. She sat on the warped wooden seat and grabbed the old ropes with both hands, using her feet to push back a little. Just like at the park when I was little, she thought. Annie felt the tight fit as her hips felt the squeeze of the swing seat and tied ropes. Billy brought out the glass of water and held the swing for Annie while she drank. When she was done Billy took the glass and placed it on the path so he would remember to take it in.

"Better?" asked Billy

"Yes, much better. I still can't believe those horses." She didn't mention the White Horses she had seen in the sea.

"Every now and then they'll come down this far but that's very unusual. You want me to push you? Maybe that will help you relax a bit."

"Okay," said Annie.

Billy started out slow.

Annie felt silly at first, but soon got into the back and forth rhythm. She was glad Billy was behind her. It made for easier conversation, as looking at him would distract her. She knew something important was coming.

"Have you and Doc talked at all about a distinction between like and want?" Billy asked in between pushes.

"No. Is that what we're going to talk about now?"

"Well, only talk if you want. I think you've had a pretty full day."

"Sure, it's okay."

Billy started right in: "If you don't know what you like, if you don't continuously touch it, feel it, play around with it, you lose it. And you know what replaces like or overtakes it?

"Want?" Annie answered with some doubt.

"Yes, want. One of the meanings of want is that of lacking something or being deficient. It's kind of like having a hole inside you that you feel needs to be filled. When your life is led by want, rather than like, it leads you to do things mindlessly or to pursue things that fill the hole, to fill the things that you think are missing. Want makes you heavy. For example, with food, you might eat without thinking. You eat to quiet your feelings instead of taking the time to feel your food, to feel how it touches what you like. But there really isn't a hole. It just feels like a hole. So after awhile you get heavier and heavier and you need more food to quiet the feelings and the cycle continues."

Annie didn't turn around. Her eyes were red and teary. Billy was describing her life—a life of want. She just wanted to swing and forget about it.

"We want what we think we lack," Billy continued, "which leads to self-judgment and invites judgment from others, which makes us feel more empty or that something is wrong with us."

"Like the hole is getting deeper," Annie chimed in. "So we keep doing the things we think we want, like eating certain kinds of food or killing ourselves at work, because we fool ourselves into believing that stuff will fill the hole."

"Exactly," said Billy.

"I've been doing that for a long time," said Annie. "It doesn't work. I'm sick of it."

"It doesn't work because there's no hole. What feels and looks like a hole is caused by ignoring the rest of yourself, the *like* part. There are no holes in you."

"So how do I get out of the hole, so to speak?" Annie asked, who began to swing herself.

"I think you know," Billy said. "You've been doing it. You touch, you feel, you play to get that part of you back, the part that is full of like. A great artist, Robert Irwin, once compared life to a swing," Billy said. "He said that you really feel that part of you that is like when are you at the top of the swing, when you can see over the wall, and see the light that is your life. But then you come back down—the real world. If you're too heavy from living a life of want, you won't be able to get back up to see and experience what you like. But if you're living a life of like, you'll be light enough so that you can push off the ground with your feet again. What you do through the entire swing matters. If you touch what's right about you and build on it, you'll like every part of the swing—you'll feel it when you push off the ground, on the way up, the most beautiful moments at the top, and then on the way down. It is about momentum. Like builds momentum. Want takes it away."

"Kind of like, like-like," Annie said, using a phrase from when she was a kid.

"Yes, like-like," said Billy, "or being childlike."

"I like that," said Annie.

And on that note, Annie gave one final, good push that sent her soaring towards the light.

Day 4

Know

Thirteen

ANNIE'S SECOND RUN

*A*nnie opened her eyes. After a few moments to adjust, she could sense that the morning light was whispering to her. Her conscious mind was telling her to fall back asleep, enjoy the comfort and luxury of the bed. The battle was on. Because her spot had been touched and was growing, her unconscious mind was suggesting otherwise, that a run on the beach to see the sunrise again might be fun. Her mind made its way back to high school, when she would rise at the crack of dawn to get in a run as part of her tennis training. She smiled. That was enough to get her to crawl out of bed. She dressed quickly, laced up her shoes, and snuck out the back.

At the entrance to the beach, she decided to unlace her shoes and take off her socks. Running barefoot on the beach was something she had always wanted to do, and today was the day.

She ventured off the path, headed toward the water line, and began to jog the two miles to the pier. She looked back every now and then just to make sure wild horses were nowhere to be found.

At age 48, Annie Jackson was re-awakening to the sound, the touch, the feel, the sight of her own life. Last night, in a brief conversation after the "swing talk," Billy had asked her, "What do you like in your life?" I like me, she answered. Billy helped her realize that's not being selfish, just the essential starting point for living. She now knew that her physical attraction to Billy was a result of her being attracted to herself, although this new realization still felt strange.

As Annie ran, everything was beginning to make sense to her. Over the years, her desire to lose weight was based on want, not like, which actually made her heavier. All Billy and Doc were doing was opening her up to what she liked, what was right about her. At first, Annie thought that playing with Billy and Doc was the cause of her reawakening. But that really wasn't the case. She was the one directing the play. But would it play in Charlottesville?

Doc put on his wraparounds and watched Annie pick up the pace near the end of her run as the big orange ball of fire lit up the beach. He watched her look out to sea, wondering what she was feeling. As Annie turned to head back to the big house, Doc waved, and Annie walked over to Billy's ramshackle home.

"So how was it going solo?" Doc asked.

"Great...super," Annie replied. "What a great way to start the day."

"How was it barefooting?" Doc asked.

"Different. Took me awhile to get adjusted."

"Do you want to sit down? asked Doc. "I've got some fresh fruit in the fridge and some homemade yogurt that Billy made. You want some?"

"That sounds heavenly," said Annie.

As Doc walked inside, Obi walked out, ball in mouth. Tail wagging, Obi made sure that Annie stroked his snout before he lay down on the deck to catch the sun's rays.

Doc returned with breakfast and Annie's taste buds came alive as she munched on the fresh strawberries and blackberries that she added to the yogurt.

"Why do things like this always taste better away from home?" Annie asked.

"Well, for one it's very fresh and usually you are somewhere where you are not in a hurry so you can eat slow to really enjoy it." Doc replied. "So what's up for today?"

"Well, I'm not sure I should tell you," said Annie, "but Sam made appointments for Kate, me, and her at the Spa for later today."

Doc did his best to remain calm.

"I know you and Billy don't like the Spa but I really feel like I need to do something with Sam since this is kind of our reunion vacation."

"That's fine," said Doc, seething inside. "I'm not the boss of you."

"You're mad. I can tell," said Annie. "What is it about the Spa that you guys despise so much?"

"Well, I think you felt it that first day. You walked out, remember?"

"Yeah, but I was all confused that first day. I don't see the harm in getting a massage, a little pampering, and maybe a little wellness coaching. Maybe it will be better than you think."

"It's not the Spa so much as what the Spa stands for," said Doc.

"What do you mean?"

Well, we went over this a little on our run."

"I don't mind hearing it again," said Annie.

"Okay, you asked for it. You like wine, right?"

"You know I do."

"I'll use the making of wine as a metaphor to explain my point."

"Okay."

"Keep in mind, I'm not a wine connoisseur," Doc said, as he leaned forward. "I'm only using it as an example to make a point."

Annie nodded.

"As I understand it, some people in the wine making business are calling for a revolution, what some call a biodynamic revolution. This is in reaction to technology that has transformed the wine industry into one of herbicides, pesticides, all sorts of chemicals that denature the vines."

"What do you mean by denatured?" asked Annie.

"That the vine no longer resembles its true nature."

"You mean vines have a true nature?" Annie asked.

"Yes, the interaction of a particular vine with soil, sun, climate is what eventually leads to each vine unfolding and flourishing in what some bio-dynamicists call the 'loveliest way possible.'"

"You're making it seem like a vine is a person," said Annie.

"Yes, exactly. We'll come back to that. But what's happened in viticulture is that because of this toxic intervention, the vine and the soil are no longer in harmony, but disharmony. Now all of the work has to occur in the wine cellar, which takes the place of nature and fabricates a good taste. The resultant wine is industrialized and artificialized."

"But the wine I drink tastes good to me," Annie said. "You're making it seem like such a bad thing."

"Well, a nice-tasting wine at what cost? No location-related quality, a wine without full self-expression, and constant intervention by the viticulturist with the pesticides, herbicides, and the aromatic yeasts added in the cellar to create a wine that at the end of the process resembles little of the original vine."

"That makes it sound really bad," said Annie.

"It is but some viticulturists are battling back. The trick, as I understand it, is to get the vines and soil back into harmony with the climate so that the vine unfolds into its full expression, to fulfill its promise."

"How does that happen?" Annie asked.

"I don't know exactly but the fascinating part, for me anyway, is that it relates to the spot, the stone Billy showed you on the beach the other day, the stone with the circles around it."

"No way," Annie said, as she leaned forward on the edge of her seat. "Tell me what you know."

"I honestly don't know," said Doc. "I'm not sure I have it right. I'm curious more than anything. But the biodynamicists say there's a spot or circle and everything starts with it, resonating outward as it grows. The spot is the entrance point, the passageway to all energy. Nothing fulfills its promise without the spot being touched and growing outward."

"Wait a second, are you talking about vines or people now?" Annie asked.

"I guess people," said Doc, who was getting tired. "But can you see how absurd it is for experts to continually intervene to change people's health behaviors or whatever? If the person is the vine, they will, over time, be moved further and further away from their own destined energies. Experts will try to save them in the cellar but by then it's too late. They can no longer grow into their promise. If they're lucky, they will end up being a nice-tasting wine."

"Geez, Doc, my head hurts," said Annie. "How did we get on this topic of wine and vines?"

"You mentioned you were going to the Spa today," said Doc.

"Right."

Annie had finished her fruit and yogurt. She was processing Doc's metaphor.

"So let me see if I'm following this," Annie said after a few moments. "Are you saying that the Spa is the wine cellar and the best it can produce is artificial wine? Is that how I would come out, an artificial wine?"

"That is precisely what I'm saying," said Doc. "People go to the Spa due to a disharmony, seeking harmony via techniques implemented by people who know about but don't really know."

"Don't know what?"

"You. To make matters worse, you yourself don't know you. I don't mean to be harsh, but a lot of health and wellness professionals use preconceived techniques and activities to make themselves feel good about what they are doing, when what they are doing is feeding into people's attempts to cope with playing The Game."

"You don't mean playing *The Game With No Name* do you?" Annie asked.

"No, playing The Game would be the antithesis of *The Game With No Name*."

"You mean like the Ladder of Success. That game?"

"Yes. It's a game people can't win no matter how much stress management, yoga, pampering, or wellness coaching you throw at them. It's like surfing in a toxic ocean.

Annie felt a little uncomfortable. She thought of her own YMCA, all of the programs and classes that were feeding The Game mentality. "I want to agree with you but I do think people feel good after these experiences, at least, what I know about my own Y and our members."

"Maybe, but it's typically a short-term feel good, and think of all of the gimmicks, the new classes, the new programs you have to keep developing to keep your members coming back—it's just old wine in new bottles, energized information instead of informed energy. Most people continue to gain weight even though they know quite a bit about what they should be doing. Do you know which generation in this country is the most obese?"

"Our kids I think," said Annie.

"Nope. It's us. The boomers," said Doc. "And we're also the group that is most knowledgeable about health and fitness. We have the information because the information is everywhere."

Annie pondered Doc's battering of her health and fitness world. "You're depressing me, Doc. I wouldn't have a clue as to how to go about changing what we're doing."

"You've been doing it at White Horse Island. You start with yourself. You get off the damn path and touch, feel, play so you really get to know what it feels like to be yourself. I know it sounds simpleton but, honestly, that's the weightless way, the way to transformative health. When you begin to live this way, you are blazing your own trail of health rather than walking on the trodden path."

"I have felt that," said Annie, being honest with her self. "And I don't know why Billy chose me but I am grateful. I feel like a changed person."

"Not a changed person," Doc corrected, "just growing into yourself. To me, that's what optimal health really means. Just do me one favor?"

"Sure, anything."

"When you go to the Spa today, weigh yourself before you do anything else." Doc was desperate. It was a stupid idea.

"Okay, but—"

"No buts, just weigh yourself. Promise."

"Okay, I promise."

The conversation had run its course for now.

"Well, thanks, Doc, for the breakfast," Annie said, as she rose to leave. "I should get going to see what Kate and Sam are up to."

"Sure, have fun at the Spa," Doc said sarcastically, as Annie began to walk away.

Without turning around, Annie lifted her arms above her head and then her two middle fingers.

Doc smiled before he rushed inside to wake Billy with the news of the pending Spa trip. Obi raised his head. His canine senses were telling him something was up.

Fourteen

The Weight of Judgment

After her shower, Annie took the DVD out of its case and ventured into the Rec room. Sipping on her orange juice, she placed the disc into the player and hit the Play button. As Annie settled into her seat, the title appeared "Annie@WHI" with a picture of a pelican gliding solo over the water in the background. She clicked on the title and immediately a quote from Charles Lindbergh about birds scrolled through in sync with a song from the Foo Fighters, a band that Maggie had introduced to her. They had become one of Annie's favorite groups.

Quickly, there appeared video snippets of pelicans flying and gliding above and near the water. Annie had never paid much attention to pelicans. They were magnificent. Annie recognized the melody and lyrics of *Learn to Fly*. After a few minutes of pelicans, Annie saw herself appear in a mix of photos that had captured her experiences so far at White Horse Island: Shooting arrows with Ian and Mac, eating Pelican Stew with Doc, running with Doc on the beach, throwing the Frisbee, playing *Turn Tennis*, body surfing with Billy, playing in the pool at the Y, and sitting on top of the dune at Jockey's Ridge. In every photo, she was deeply engaged in an activity or smiling. Her favorite was the one with her talking to the kids while they played in the sand. The music seemed to be perfectly in sync with the photos that flashed through. Annie lost herself in the music and photos, which ended with a picture of her laughing while standing around the firepit and watching Billy stir his Pelican Stew.

"There you are?" said Kate as she walked in to the Rec room. "What are you watching?"

"You won't believe this," said Annie. "I'm just blown away by it. Come watch it with me."

Kate snuggled up on the couch with her coffee as Annie hit Play again.

When it ended, Kate asked: "Where did you get this?"

"It was in the FedEx package delivered last night," Annie replied.

"It's incredible," said Kate. "But who put it together?"

"I have no idea," said Annie. "It can't be Billy or Doc or Harry because they're in some of the pictures."

"Let's watch it again," said Kate.

This time Annie was able to connect some of the lyrics to the photos. Whoever put this together knew exactly what they were doing.

"What does that mean? 'Make my way back home when I learn to fly,'" asked Kate.

Yeah, I picked up on that, too," said Annie. "Maybe home is my spot and all of this has been about learning to fly, so to speak, so I can get back to my home, to being myself."

"Well, I'm jealous. I would watch this every night. It's great," said Kate.

Both Annie and Kate missed the line "Hook me up a new revolution 'cause this one is a lie."

The white, unmarked van pulled up to the Spa. The driver was a good-looking guy with broad shoulders and long, silver hair. A smaller man wearing wraparound shades was riding shotgun. Dressed in brown uniforms that were misfit, both men got out with the small guy grabbing a box out of the back. As planned, they walked into the Spa with the silver-haired delivery man in the lead.

"Hello, beautiful," the man said.

"May I help you?" said the young, blonde receptionist without looking up from her riveting reading of *People* magazine.

"Yes, we're technicians with the *Weightless Weigh* Company," said the silver-haired man. "We have a package to deliver."

"I don't think we're expecting any deliv—" as she looked up and caught the man's eyes piercing her soul. "Uh…I'm sorry…what did you say?"

The man flashed a smile. "We have a package to deliver. We have an order here to replace the weight scale in the women's locker room with this newer model." The smaller guy lifted the box for the woman to see.

"Oh…uh…okay…I'll take it. Do I need to sign for anything?" the woman asked, still spellbound by the man's eyes.

"No, beautiful, but the orders here say that we need to remove the old scale and replace it with the new one. There were complaints of the scale being inaccurate. We're replacing the older model with the state-of-the-art *WW-Three Sixty.*"

"Well, I hadn't heard of any—"

"We could use your help, beautiful. Please come with us to show us the women's locker room and make sure it's empty. That way we can make the switch and calibrate the new scale. It will only take a few minutes."

Mesmerized by the man's voice and those eyes, the disinterested young blonde who talked with Annie was now very interested in helping. She led the men through the fake waterfall, down the tiled hall, and to the back. "Wait here," she said as she walked in the locker room, coming out seconds later. "It's all clear. Are you sure you don't need me to help in there?"

"You've been plenty helpful already, beautiful. We'll just be a couple of minutes. Just stand guard for us."

The blonde smiled and nodded, feeling good that she was actually doing something useful.

Harry and Doc walked in and quickly got to work. Doc took the new scale from the box and placed it next to the old one. He grabbed the old one and put it in the box.

"Are you sure this is going to work?" asked Harry.

"Well, Ian and Mac are engineers. I have to trust that they knew what they were doing with the calibration," Doc said.

"Again, why are you purposefully putting an inaccurate scale in the women's locker room?" asked Harry.

"Annie is coming later. She's going to weigh herself and I want her to believe that she has already lost weight."

"Why? Isn't that cheating?"

"Harry, I don't have time to explain all of this," Doc said, as he took off his shoes and hopped on the scale, which illuminated "145" in bright, digital numbers.

Ever the scientist, Doc needed corroboration of the five pounds differential.

"Hey, swimmers, are usually pretty anal with their weight, right?"

"Yeah," said Harry.

"How much do you weigh?"

"One ninety five," Harry proudly proclaimed.

"Okay, take off your shoes and step up on there."

Harry obeyed Doc's order. The scale read "190."

"Perfect," said Doc, as he picked up the box. "Let's get out of here."

As Harry opened the door, the blonde was talking with a couple of older women in white robes and slippers, waiting to enter. "Okay, ladies, they're done. You can go in now," she said.

The two women hesitated as they caught a glimpse of Harry, and then walked in as Harry held the door, nodding and giving the women a quick wink.

"Thanks, beautiful. We appreciate the help," Harry said to the blonde, as he and Doc hurried towards the entrance. "There's no charge for this. That scale was malfunctioning and under warranty."

"Okay, well thanks," said the receptionist, who stood in the foyer waving as Harry and Doc got back in the van and drove away.

T he three women had made it out to the beach and were enjoying the sun and solitude, which had been the master plan for the reunion week before the vacation had been interrupted by Annie's caseworkers. Sam had apologized to Annie that morning, followed by a hug. Annie didn't tell Sam or Kate about her like vs. want conversation with Billy. She didn't feel they were ready to hear about it and she wasn't sure she understood the distinction well enough to talk about it.

They took turns guessing who had put together Annie's personalized music video—a mystery man, Ian and Mac, maybe Chrissie—but none of those guesses rang true to Annie. Annie had let Sam watch the DVD later that morning. Even she admitted it was pretty good, although she found it creepy that someone was taking pictures of Annie without her knowledge.

Sam's cell rang, announcing a new text. "Shit," she said, after reading a few lines. "Some crap happening at work that needs my attention. I've got to go in and get on my laptop to put out some fires."

"Sam, don't they know you're on vacation," said Kate.

"Hey, the world of marketing never sleeps," said Sam. "We've got about an hour before we go to the Spa. Come and get me if I'm not out in time."

"Will do," said Annie, who had been close to napping.

Annie and Kate watched Sam walk back to the house.

"I can't believe Sam's figure," said Annie. "I mean her body looks like a fit woman in her mid twenties. How does she do it?"

"Well, no kids," said Kate. "She's got time. She's got access to a fitness center at work and their on-site cafeteria has healthy food options. Shall I go on?"

"No, I get it. But I was more fit than Sam in high school. I guess I'm still using that as my reference point.

"You mean a judgment point," said a voice behind them.

"Doc, I know that's you," said Annie, who didn't need to turn around to confirm her suspicions. "Can't you let me process the wine stuff before you hit me with something new. I mean, my spot needs a little room to breathe, you know."

"I can come back later," said Doc, who promptly sat down in the sand near their blankets.

"No, that's fine," said Annie, who sat up and turned to face Doc. Kate did the same. "What do you mean by judgment point?"

"Well, I've got something for you to read. It's from a book. It's only 400 words so you can read it quick. Kate, I brought one for you too," said Doc, as he handed each of them the one page brief.

"Just read it and then I want to hear your reaction," Doc said.

After a few minutes, Kate was the first to react: "I'm adventurous but this is totally irresponsible. It makes me a little angry. It seems almost sexist."

"I'm envious," said Annie. "His life is so exciting compared to mine. He's obviously a famous musician."

"Okay, Doc, what's the point?" asked Kate.

"Wait a minute," said Annie. "I want to know who this is. Is it Billy Joel?"

My Life
(In Four Hundred Words or Less)

I flunked out of college. I learned to play the guitar, lived on the beach, lived in the French Quarter, finally got laid, and didn't go to Vietnam. I got back into school, started a band, got a job on Bourbon Street, graduated from college, flunked my draft physical, broke up my band, and went on the road solo. I signed a record deal, got married, moved to Nashville, had my guitars stolen, bought a Mercedes, worked at Billboard magazine, put out my first album, went broke, met Jerry Jeff Walker, wrecked the Mercedes, got divorced, and moved to Key West. I sang and worked on a fishing boat, went totally crazy, did a lot of dope, met the right girl, made another record, had a hit, bought a boat, and sailed away to the Caribbean. I started another band, worked the road, had my second and last hit, bought a house in Aspen, started spending summers in New England, got married, broke my leg three times in one year, had a baby girl, made more records, bought a bigger boat, and sailed away to St. Barts. I got separated from the right girl, sold the boat, sold the house in Aspen, moved back to Key West, worked the road, and made more records. I rented an apartment in Paris, went to Brazil for Carnival, learned to fly, went into therapy, quit doing dope, bought my first seaplane, flew over the Caribbean, almost got a second divorce, moved to Malibu for more therapy, and got back with the right girl. I worked the road, moved back to Nashville, took off in an F-14 from an aircraft carrier, bought a summer home on Long Island, had another baby girl. I found the perfect seaplane and moved back to Florida. Cameron Marley joined me in the house of women. I built a home on Long Island, crashed the perfect seaplane in Nantucket, lived through it thanks to Navy training, tried to slow down a little, woke up one morning and I was looking at fifty, trying to figure out what comes next.

Doc laughed. "Hardly," thinking about Joel's short-lived marriage to a college student who had once sat in his class. "I'll tell you in a minute but the point as I see it is that you both immediately judged either this guy or yourself."

"What do you mean?" asked Kate. "Kate, you immediately judged him as irresponsible, and, Annie, you judged yourself and your own life based on his."

"I judged myself?" asked Annie.

"Yeah," said Kate, "you said you were 'envious.'"

"Aren't you?" asked Annie.

"Heck no, I think he went way over the line as far as adventure goes," replied Kate.

"Okay, so I'm a little jealous of this guy's life. I guess I'm not sure why that is a big deal. This doesn't seem to connect with me, Doc, like some of the other things we've been doing."

Doc hoped Annie was ready for this. They had started with what's right about her. He was hoping that was enough to be a buffer. "Can I be frank in front of Kate?" Doc asked.

"Sure, she's my best friend," said Annie. Kate nodded.

"The main reason you're overweight is because you judge yourself or invite judgment from others," Doc said. "All of the judgment is just weighing you down."

Annie was now paying close attention, not sure whether to recoil from or embrace what Doc was saying.

"I'm not really aware that I do that," said Annie, unsure of what else to say.

"I think you are," said Doc. "All the weight, the baggage, the walls push in on your spot, making you feel heavy, tired, lacking energy. It's why you slouch, it's why you don't play with Dylan or John or your staff or your members."

"But I feel like I'm changing. I've felt different since I've been here," said Annie.

"It's not really about changing. Lots of people try to change by going on diets, but when you go on a diet or listen to the expert nutritionist, you are exchanging one set of baggage for another. You are inviting judgment because you are now on someone else's path. And that judgment by you or from others weighs you down further. That's why you've been gaining weight over the years, *even when* trying to lose weight."

"But don't you have to give up some things to lose weight?" asked Kate.

"NO!" Doc exclaimed, as he stood up and started pacing, kicking the sand in various directions.

Doc's behavior, which was out of character, made Annie and Kate a little nervous.

"Can't you see what's right in front of you," Doc implored, trying to gather himself. "You can't become something by giving up something. Annie has built walls around her original nature, her spot. Those walls are weighing her down. She's not living her true nature so she doesn't move her body or eat foods that feed that nature. It's a withering on the vine."

"Annie, do you know what in the hell Doc is talking about?" asked Kate.

"Sort of," said Annie, who finally realized that Doc was talking as much about himself as he was about her. She stood up and put her arm around Doc. He started to sob.

"Is that what happened to you, Doc?" Annie asked.

Doc nodded, unable to speak. Annie patted his back for reassurance.

"What happened, Doc?" asked Kate. "What happened to you?"

"I let go of my dreams, my aspirations," said Doc. "Actually I gave myself up to academe, which was against my true nature."

"Well, how come you didn't gain weight?" Kate asked.

Doc was more controlled now. "Sorry about the outburst. I guess the best way to answer your question, Kate, is that we all gain weight in different ways. My weight gain was an autoimmune disease that I now have to deal with for the rest of my life."

"So what's the punch line to all of this, Doc?" asked Annie.

"Well, I would say instead of giving up something, become some-thing," Doc said. That's how we lose weight. You'll experience and *know* how it feels to be yourself rather than knowing about something, not really experiencing it."

"Doc, I honestly believe I have started to do that. And you and Billy have helped me. You've got to believe that."

Doc nodded.

"Hey, Annie, we need to get going to get Sam and head over to the Spa," Kate said.

Doc winced.

"Oh, right. You going to be all right, Doc?" Annie asked as she began gathering up the beach paraphernalia with Kate.

Doc nodded.

"So who is the guy that wrote the four hundred words?" asked Kate.

"Jimmy Buffett," said Doc. "A modern day pirate."

"I do like him," said Kate. "But I still think he stepped over the line a few times."

Doc shrugged. Freeing oneself from judgment could be as difficult as escaping a rip tide. He watched them walk away and noticed that Annie's shoulders were rolled back the way nature had designed them. He smiled away the few tears his condition had allowed and walked back to the shack, humming the tune from "Margaritaville."

Fifteen

TRIP TO THE SPA

From Annie's pirate perch on the deck high atop the beach, she performed a 270-degree scan. Nothing. No one on the swing. No one on the shack's deck. No Doc. No Billy. No Obi. No *Game With No Name* players. Just a few vacationers spotting the beach like polka dots on a summer dress. In some ways, she was glad. She needed a respite from their relentlessness. Annie felt she needed a relax, refresh, rejuvenate spa experience with her best friends. She didn't want to bump into Doc or Billy on the way to the Spa as they might try to talk her out of going.

"Okay, guys, coast is clear," Annie yelled in to the house, feeling a little guilty. "Let's go."

Kate and Sam joined her on the deck and once they got below they headed to the path that would take them past the shack to the Spa. Music was playing inside the shack. Annie recognized "Margaritaville."

"Hurry up, " she whispered. All three picked up the pace and then slowed once they passed the shack.

"Hey look," said Sam, "it's high tide." The water was coming up near the path. The three women stopped to watch. A couple of surfers were playing in the waves, but Annie was more interested in the white caps.

As the waves crested into the white foam, they morphed into the White Horses rising out of the water. Annie looked at Sam and Kate, who seemed to be following a pod of pelicans skimming the water. Do they see them? she wondered.

"What are you guys watching?" Annie asked.

"The pelicans," replied Kate.

"You don't see anything else?" asked Annie.

"No, why do you see something?" asked Kate.

"No," Annie said. "Just curious."

The White Horses kept rising out of the crests and galloping toward her. "Come play, Annie," the horses whispered just before they disappeared into the sand.

"Billy?" Billy? Is that you?" Annie asked, in a soft voice.

"What?" asked Sam. "Did you say Billy's name?"

"Annie…Annie, you just asked for Billy," said Kate, rubbing Annie's arm in an attempt to awaken her from her white horse fixation.

"Uh…oh…no I didn't," Annie replied, flustered.

"Yes, you did," said Sam. "That man has some hold on you."

"It's all right, Annie, you were day dreaming," said Kate. "Let's get to the Spa.

"Yes, let's get to the Spa," said Annie, while looking out to the ocean. Only the surfers were playing in the water. The White Horses were gone.

Annie was relieved that they reached the Spa with no further incidents. She had mentally prepared herself to squelch the negative feelings she experienced during her brief visit earlier in the week. Sam checked them in with the blonde receptionist for their two-hour Relax, Refresh, Rejuvenate session. Annie was getting the wellness coaching session as a bonus, paid for by Sam and Kate.

The whiteness was almost blinding. She still felt out of place, even more so. Her mind wandered to the White Horses. She wanted to run away with them, to escape the Spa experience, but she didn't.

A pasty woman shuffled them back to the locker room and told them how to get to their private suites to begin their session. She handed each woman a key for her lockers. Once inside the pristine locker room, Annie felt a rush of embarrassment as she took her clothes off in preparation for the robe and slippers.

As she bent over to take off her shoes, she spotted the WW-360 in the corner and remembered Doc's admonition about weighing herself. As she cautiously stepped on the scale, she noticed that it looked very similar to the one in her Charlottesville YMCA. A "143" popped up, which surprised Annie. She quickly stepped off and then tried again. Again, "143." That's five pounds less than what I weighed when I left for White Horse Island, thought Annie.

"How's it looking, Annie?" asked Kate.

"Oh, not bad," replied Annie, not wanting to get into a discussion with Kate and Sam about her weight.

Annie and Kate put on their swimsuits and then the robe and slippers. Annie noticed that Sam was naked under the robe.

"Okay, ladies, let's go have some fun," said Sam, as she opened a door that led to some chairs and a small pool.

"Look at these chairs," said Kate. "Aren't they cool."

"I think they're tepidarium chairs," said Annie. "They warm from the inside."

"Let's try them," said Sam.

They each sat in one and the feeling for Annie was instant pleasure. She took a deep breath, held it, and slowly exhaled. She felt her body relax.

"This is wonderful," said Kate.

Annie was too relaxed to speak, the warmth oozing through her entire body.

After a few minutes, Annie forced herself off the chair and gently eased her body into the spacious warm pool. More pleasure. Kate and Sam followed. She was envious of their bodies but reminded herself that somehow she had lost five pounds. Maybe Doc and Billy are right, she thought. As they were drying off with the Spa towels, the locker room attendant, dressed in an all-white outfit, notified them that they're rooms and therapists were ready. After re-robing, they followed the attendant out of the pool area to a bevy of separate rooms.

"See you girls after," said Sam, who smiled at her male therapist.

"Have fun," said Kate.

Annie waved to them and walked into her private suite.

As Annie soaked in the hydrotherapy tub, she had to admit that her therapist, Lisa, had been quite good. She had dry brushed the dead skin cells, and then scrubbed Annie's skin with an oil that furthered the exfoliation process. Annie then rinsed in the shower and came back for her deep tissue, full body massage, enhanced by a renewing herbal oil. After the massage, Lisa wrapped Annie's body in some kind of herbal goop that Lisa told her was guaranteed to detox and rejuvenate. Covered in plastic, warm blankets, and heated towels, Annie had 30 minutes to herself.

During the body wrap, Annie's mind had wandered to the day she met John. She had been at the UVa tennis courts practicing her serve at one of the far courts when a guy had walked up and just started watching her, which was a little disconcerting. Annie started missing serves.

"Pretty good," said the guy, as Annie was gathering up the balls, "but if you arch your back a bit more, you'll get a little more power."

"Really," said Annie. "Thanks for the tip."

"Do you want to hit for awhile?" the guy asked. "It doesn't look my partner is going to show."

"Okay," said Annie.

"I'm, John," the guy said.

"Annie. Nice to meet you. Do you go to school here?"

"Yeah, I'm a management major. I'm a sophomore."

"Me too," said Annie. "Social work."

John was an excellent hitting partner. He was very fast and could hit with good power for a guy that was no bigger than she was. One thing led to another and after that first day, just like that, Annie and John were inseparable.

How did we become separable? Annie wondered.

Lisa came back and finished off the full body experience with a full-scalp massage using some kind of pink mud combined with a peppermint-smelling oil. Annie's entire head felt tingly afterwards as she rinsed off again. Lisa had then led her to the hydrotherapy room, where she could soak for 20 minutes in a copper tub that Lisa claimed could provide relief for weary muscles, arthritis, and headaches.

"Here's some antioxidant rich green tea," said Lisa as she planted the cup on the tub's ledge and headed for the door.

"Thank you," said Annie, as she leaned her head back to rest on a soft, white towel that Lisa had placed at the head of the tub.

Annie took a few sips of the tea, and moments later felt an intoxicating rush of what she could only describe as intimacy. Annie closed her eyes. In her mind's eye, the White Horses appeared. "Come play, Annie," they whispered. Then Billy and Doc appeared, riding the White Horses as they rose out of the sea.

"Annie, watch out for 'What are your goals?'" Doc said.

"Watch out for 'What do you want to change?'" said Billy. "Those are 'know about' questions generated by experts on the path."

Then others appeared on the horses. "Remember, *Turn Tennis*, Annie. Feel it," said Chrissie, brandishing her tennis racket like a trident.

Ian and Mac appeared, waving their hats like cowboys riding wild broncos. "You've got your own data, Annie, trust it."

Handsome Harry was next, holding a bag of Serenity Now: "What's your *Easy Speed*, Annie? How do you want to feel today?"

Even the FedEx guy showed up, holding his arrow: "Once you feel it, it's always there, Annie."

She saw Obi sitting on one of the White Horses, ball in mouth, wagging his tail.

In the moment just before Annie opened her eyes, she felt it: a moment where there was nothing, where "noise" gives way to silence, being "full" gives way to space, and "busy" slows down to stillness. In that moment of silence, space, and stillness, her spot, which had been buried by years of judgment burst through those walls. As she opened her eyes, Annie felt a rush of energy pulsate through her body. She had a powerful urge to move, to get out of the Spa, to run. It was a transcendent moment.

Not sure of exactly what to do, Annie got out of the tub, hurriedly dried herself, put her swimsuit on, threw the robe over her, and stepped into the slippers.

Lisa arrived as Annie was leaving.

"Oh, you're done," said Lisa, surprised. "You've got a few minutes before your coaching session. I can take you back to the locker room."

"I...I...I just realized I have another appointment," said Annie, as she moved quickly towards the door. "I'll have to reschedule."

"Oh, Okay," said Lisa. "I'll tell Coach Meg."

"Thanks," said Annie. "I can find my way out."

Annie burst through the door, and performed her best race walk imitation down the hall. Nearing the locker room, she caught up to Sam and Kate. As she rushed by them, she reached into the robe pocket, grabbed the key, and threw it over her shoulder. "GET MY CLOTHES FOR ME," she yelled, continuing down the hall.

Kate caught the perfect toss.

"ANNIE, ARE YOU CRAZY? WHERE ARE YOU GOING?" shouted Sam.

"What in the hell?" asked Kate, as both she and Sam started to run after Annie, clogging down the hall in their slippers.

As Annie entered the foyer, she flung off her robe and slippers and left them in her wake on the pristine floor.

"Ma'am, what are you doing?" asked the blonde receptionist. "Did you pay for the services?"

Annie opened the door and stepped on the path just as Kate and Sam reached the foyer. She leaped onto the sand and broke into a sprint, heading toward the White Horses. She felt free. She finally knew what free felt like.

Sam and Kate knew they would not be able to catch her. Sam picked up the robe and slippers and handed them to the stunned receptionist as they headed back to the locker room.

Two older women who were waiting in the foyer for their Spa appointment had watched Annie's mad dash. "Wow," said one of the women to her friend. "I hope my massage is as good as hers."

Annie followed the call of the White Horses, which was loudest as she approached Billy's shack. She veered left toward the water and smashed into the waves, driving and lifting her legs like a hurdler. A few strides outs, she dove in and started swimming out into the waves, to play with the White Horses. Going by feel, she swam effortlessly until what seemed like a reasonable stopping point. When Annie stood up, she took a moment to catch her bearings, trying to fathom what she had just done. It was all a blur. Did I just run out of the Spa in my bathing suit? she asked herself. She looked in to the shore and saw what looked like Billy and Doc sitting on the shack's deck. She waved enthusiastically. The two men waved back as Annie bobbed in the water.

"Well, that was interesting," said Doc, referring to Annie's run along the beach and dive into the water. "She either loved the Spa and is feeling renewed or hated it and couldn't wait to get out of there."

"I'm guessing Lisa gave Annie the green tea that I brewed," said Billy.

"Do you think it's ethical to give her one of your homemade concoctions?" Doc asked.

"It's all natural," said Billy. "No harm, no foul. And look who's talking, you're the one who came up with the idea of planting a weightless scale at the Spa."

"Touché," said Doc. "Man, that place gives me the creeps. What does your green tea do?"

"Let's just say it brings out one's natural inclinations," replied Billy.

"You mean to run like hell out of the Spa and dive headlong into the ocean?" Doc asked.

"More or less."

"To change the topic a little, I've been reading this book *Born to Run*. It confirms what we know in an indirect way in that the journalist makes a direct connection to finding himself in running and being attracted to *lighter* foods." He didn't go on a diet, he just naturally became more interested in eating foods that created energy and made him feel light. And he lost weight, slept better, and, of course, ran better."

"What's your point?" Billy asked. "You already know this."

"Well, how does this happen?" asked Doc. "I mean, I know it happens. I've experienced it myself and I know you have as well. But how does it happen?"

"Basically, you go from *knowing about* things, to *knowing* things," Billy said. "When you start paying attention, taking the time to figure out and experience what you like, playing around, you begin to truly *know* things. When you settle based on want, you *know about* things, which is a much weaker way of experiencing things."

"So, if I'm following you, Annie is making strides with losing weight because she is beginning to know things as she awakens that clean, unspoiled spot through touch, feel, play. This makes her feel lighter, which attracts her to activities that naturally connect with that feeling, things like physical activity and foods that feed that energy source—informed energy."

"Yes," said Billy.

"But how does that happen exactly?" asked Doc.

"It's not really necessary to know how it happens," replied Billy. "But if you pushed me I would say it relates to the battle that goes on inside between the conscious and the unconscious mind."

"Okay, now we're getting somewhere," said Doc, as he leaned forward to hear Billy's explanation.

"Speaking of unconscious and conscious, here come Sam and Kate," said Billy.

Doc turned towards the path to see the two women striding with a purpose, making a beeline towards the two men.

"Hey, guys," said Kate. "Have you seen Annie?"

Billy pointed out to sea. Annie was motioning for them to come join her in the waves.

"What happened at the Spa?" asked Doc.

"That's what we're trying to figure out," said Sam, looking suspiciously at Billy. "Annie just bolted out of the Spa. Didn't even stay for her wellness coaching."

"Too bad," said Doc.

"Came to her senses I suppose," said Billy. "Why don't you just go play with Annie. Have some real fun for a change instead of some fake, artificial fun like at the Spa."

"Oh, you would just love that, wouldn't you, Mr. touchy feely," said Sam.

"Sam, let's just go play with Annie," said Kate, who really didn't like the direction the conversation was going. "Billy and Doc had nothing to do with this."

"Oh yes they did," said Sam. "They're ruining this whole vacation, with their interruptions and stupid games. Life detectives, my ass."

"You don't really want to get into this with us," said Billy.

Doc wasn't sure if he liked being included in what was heading for a major confrontation.

"Like I told you last night," said Billy, "I don't think you're a very good friend to Annie. You're imposing your guilt and judgment onto her and it's weighing her down. Why do you do that?"

"You egotistical, self-help hack," said Sam. "What, you couldn't make it in medicine so you just hole up in this dirty, old shack, pretending to be Mr. cool to attract women like Annie."

"Answer the question, why do you do that?" Billy persisted.

"Do what?" asked Sam.

"Why do you pretend to be Annie's friend all these years when it's more about you than her. I bet I know."

"You don't know shit," said Sam.

"You slept with John, didn't you," Billy said.

Sam took a step back. Kate dropped her clothes bag. Doc coughed, leaned back, and almost fell over.

"You're nuts," said Sam, after taking a moment to collect herself.

"Am I?" asked Billy. "You're whole life has been about using sex to fill a hole from the shadow of some trauma you could never escape. I bet you fucked John and then sent him Annie's way because he didn't measure up to your fuckability standards. You sent him to Annie as a way to feel your superiority over her. So what's the truth: did you fuck John before or after he met Annie?"

Sam was beet red. "I don't have to stand here and listen to these ridiculous accusations," Sam said, trying to deflect the truth. "C'mon, Kate, let's go."

"Uh…Uhmmm…I think I'll maybe go join Annie in the water," said Kate.

"Suit yourself," huffed Sam, as she turned and headed towards the rental house. Doc and Billy couldn't help themselves as they watched Sam wiggle away.

Doc looked at Billy. Billy gave a nod and Doc rose to rush inside the shack. It was time to get Harry back in action.

"Excuse me," Doc said to Kate, as he left to call Harry.

"Sorry about that," said Billy to Kate, who was still dumbfounded by what had just occurred. "But I just couldn't let her get away with her high and mighty anymore. My job is to help Annie lose weight. Sam is an obstacle."

Kate slumped down in Doc's chair. "I'm just at a loss," she said. "I really don't know what's going on. Sam is my friend too. I've always suspected something was up between her and John. Sam always acts weird around him. And she did screw my ex-boyfriend in high school so I wouldn't put it past her.

"So you believe I'm right?" asked Billy.

"Yes, although I don't know why. I hardly know you and I don't know how you figured it out."

"That is what I do. Clues were everywhere."

"What should I do with Annie?" asked Kate.

"Just continue to be her friend, like you always have," Billy replied.

"But do I...you know...tell her?" asked Kate.

"I don't think so," said Billy. "I think Sam might confess once she comes to grips with the truth."

"I think I need a swim in the ocean with my best friend," said Kate. "Is it okay if I leave my stuff here?"

"Sure."

As Kate was walking away, she turned back to Billy. "You know, I still don't understand all of this. And I don't get why or how you are working with Annie on losing weight. It's the weirdest weight loss program I've ever seen. But I do know Annie has been more playful than I can remember and she's smiling a lot. So, I guess, thanks."

Billy nodded and watched as Kate ran to join her friend.

*K*ate swam out to meet Annie.

"Kate the Great," said Annie.

"Hello, Annie Oakley, said Kate.

"Aren't these waves awesome," said Annie. "Just perfect for body surfing. I'm going to come out tomorrow morning. You want to come out with me?"

"Sure," said Kate, as they both bobbed in the waves.

"Where did Sam go?" asked Annie.

"Uh...well...she went back to the house. She was a little tired," said Kate.

"Oh, too bad. I was going to teach her some body surfing moves," said Annie. "Are you ready to try it?"

"Yeah, but before we do I was wondering what in the world happened to you in the Spa?" asked Kate.

"Oh, well, all I remember is that I was laying in the therapy tub. I drank some green tea and I just started having these visions, maybe they were hallucinations, I don't really know. Then, I had this powerful urge to run. So that's what I did."

"But you realize that you ran through the Spa and then just threw off your robe in the foyer," said Kate.

"That part is a little fuzzy," said Annie. "I'm sorry if I embarrassed you guys. But I just had to get out of there and run to the ocean."

"But couldn't you have changed your clothes first?" asked Kate.

"I guess, but the White Horses were whispering to me to come play."

"Oh my God!" said Kate.

"What, what," said Annie, who swallowed some of the salt water and tried to expectorate.

"Did you see White Horses in the water when we were walking to the Spa?" asked Kate.

"Yes…yes," said Annie, in between spits. "I've been dreaming about them and they have appeared in these visions I've been having ever since I arrived. Did you see them?"

"Yes, but I didn't want to say anything because I thought you guys would think I'm nuts," said Kate. "But I've only seen them that one time. You've seen them more than that?"

"Yes," said Annie.

"Weird," said Kate. "What do you think it means?"

"I don't know. But I'd be willing to bet that there's some connection with Billy."

"Wow," said Kate, "This is some weight loss program you're in."

Annie smiled and began to teach Kate how to body surf.

Sixteen

PELICAN'S PRINCIPLES

*D*oc walked out of the shack to inform Billy that Harry was on the case. He put on his wraparounds and petted Obi. He was dressed for a run.

"Going running?" Billy asked.

"Yep, unless you want to talk more about the conscious and unconscious?"

"It's simple, really," said Billy.

"To you, maybe," said Doc as he sat down.

"If you look at Annie," Billy began, "she was taught, like most of us, a conscious model of learning and doing, thinking your way through things, learning when and how to use and control emotions, and so forth. We then try to make connections between our thoughts and feelings and our behavior. Who taught Annie this model?"

"Her parents, teachers, coaches," Doc responded quickly.

"Right, people who cared about her, hopefully. So if she follows these models taught by these experts that she cares about she gets approval from them and feels good about herself."

"I think I know where you're going with this," said Doc.

"Where?" asked Billy.

"Well, if these people only know about and don't really know now Annie is just doing things to get approval, and these things might not be very useful for improving or getting better."

"That's part of it. They can only take you so far because we know that the best performances involve more than the conscious mind. They involve a level of engagement and processing that is much deeper and richer than the conscious mind can deliver. But most of us cling to the conscious model because it is what we have been taught and we don't want to feel shame or inadequacy when we let down the people who love us by rejecting their how of doing things."

"So that's why Annie has gained weight all these years," Doc said excitedly. "It's the judgment thing. All of this worry, fear, and shame just weigh her down."

"Let's take it further," said Billy. "What if these engaging, high performing moments are, in fact, driven by a process outside of the thoughts and feelings we have been taught under the model of approval and judgment?"

"The unconscious," Doc said.

Billy nodded and leaned forward. "The people I've worked with have another model whispering to them, tugging at them, and they have the courage and the will to listen and to act. And in the process, they experience a transcendence of themselves."

"They touch, feel, and play," Doc said, affirming the process that Annie had been experiencing.

"Yes, and through that process, they begin to know, trust, and create their own lives, their own performances. But this part is as difficult as the touch, feel, and play because the world we live in doesn't readily acknowledge the unconscious gift of our minds. Few people do this...and almost no one who is really good doesn't do this."

"Annie is doing this. I know it," said Doc. "Eureka, I feel like running naked on the beach," said Doc.

"Please don't," said Billy.

"But now I know why I always get a nauseating reaction to the health behavior change approach—change your thoughts and feelings to change your behavior, blah, blah, blah. If how and when we move or what and when we eat are driven by unconscious processes that are brought to life when that clean, unspoiled spot is touched and reawakened, trying to change thoughts and feelings that are mostly irrelevant anyway will fail—totally and completely."

"You da man," said Billy.

"That's how the *Born to Run* guy that I was telling you about earlier started eating better. He made the unconscious conscious."

"You could look at it that way," Billy said. "Or maybe he aligned the two models, merged them into one."

"Is that possible?" asked Doc.

"Why not?"

Doc stood up. He had had a moment of clarity, a transcendent moment.

"C'mon, Obi," Doc said. Obi perked up. Ball in mouth. Ready.

"Where ya going?" Billy asked.

"I don't know, I'm just going." Doc started running towards the water line with Obi running after him.

Billy watched until Doc and Obi disappeared into the surf and sand. He spotted Annie and Kate who were still body surfing amidst the White Horses. Billy Pelican closed his eyes. He thought of his grandfather and the White Horses, the basketball hoop at the Whalehead Club, the crazy night when he almost lost his life, the many twists and turns his life had taken. He was thankful for it all. Billy opened his eyes and went inside to check on dinner.

Exhausted from the bodysurfing, Kate and Annie were slowly gathering up Kate's bags full of clothes she had left on the deck of Billy's shack.

"Have you been inside yet?" Kate asked, snapping her head towards the shack.

"No," said Annie.

"Should we?" asked Kate.

"Should we go in?" asked Annie.

"Yeah, why not, take a look around," said Kate. "Aren't you a little curious as to how your case worker lives. Plus, something smells awfully good."

"What if they're in there?" asked Annie.

"We saw Doc running with Obi, remember," said Kate. "We'll knock, and if Billy answers we'll think of some kind of excuse."

"I guess," said Annie.

Kate dropped the bags, walked to the sliding glass door and screen and peered in. "Hello," she called out. She knocked on the glass door that was pulled to the side. No answer. Kate slid open the screen door and they stepped inside.

A tiny kitchen greeted them with a big pot of something simmering on the stove—the source of the smell. A quick perusal suggested that the inside was as shack-like as the outside.

Books and magazines were scattered everywhere—on the floor, on shelves, on the couch, which was the only place to sit other than two rickety chairs around the small kitchen table. Tins of skoal were also lying around. Two small bedrooms were off the living room, which was about the size of the kitchen. That was the extent of the shack.

"How can he live like this?" whispered Kate.

"You don't need to whisper, Kate, there's no one here," said Annie.

"Look, he has a bike," said Kate, pointing to the Trek in the corner of the living room. "But there's no TV."

"Let's get out of here," said Annie. "Billy could walk in any second."

Kate nodded. As they turned to leave, Annie spotted a small corkboard near the sliding door entrance with a lone note drawn on legal paper held up by a stickpin.

"What's this?" she asked, pointing to the note.

As they moved closer, Annie could see "Pelican's Principles."

"Let me see," said Kate as she moved closer to the board.

"This is some kind of life philosophy," said Kate.

"Yeah, I recognize some of the principles from what I've been doing the past few days," said Annie. "But some of them I have no clue—'Goals come later, if at all'? What's that mean?"

"I'm not sure," said Kate. "Why are these called 'Pelican's Principles'?" asked Kate.

"Oh, that's Billy nickname, Billy Pelican," Annie said.

"That's a great name," said Kate, chuckling. "What's his real name?"

"Billy Hamilton. Let's get out of here," said Annie, as she tried to memorize the rest of the list.

Pelican's Principles
No real order but all important for losing weight

- *You do not feel what you do not touch*
- *You start with what's right about you*
- *Feel, not feelings*
- *Play to discover your gifts that turn into skills*
- *Goals come later, if at all*
- *Freedom is what you feel in action*
- *You probably won't like the things you want*
- *You can't choose what you don't know*
- *Take what you like into the world*
- *Trust is the foundation for doing well what is worth doing*
- *We want what we think we lack, which invites judgment*
- *What you like about your life will heal you*
- *Life is a single, multilayered task*
- *Informed energy fuels the feel*

As they moved toward the door, Annie couldn't help herself. She lifted the lid off the cooking pot and used the lid to waft the steam toward her nose as she leaned over the pot. She inhaled to take it all in. Pelican stew, she thought, damn that smells good.

"C'mon Annie," said Kate, who was already on the deck.

Annie replaced the lid, took a quick look around, and left the shack with the *Pelican's Principles* burning in her brain and the Pelican Stew wreaking havoc on her stomach.

Annie and Kate plopped down on the sofa. What a day.

"I'm pooped," said Kate.

"Me too," said Annie. "I think I'm just staying in tonight."

"Fine with me," said Kate. "But what are we going to eat? I'm famished."

"Good question. Maybe there is some take out place nearby," said Annie, as her mind floated to the Pelican Stew.

"Let's take showers and regroup," said Kate.

"Good plan," said Annie.

Kate spotted the note on the coffee table that had been used for experimenting with *Serenity Now*:

> Kate and Annie,
>   I went out with Harry. Don't wait up for me. Let's do something fun tomorrow.
>   Sam

Kate was kind of glad as she handed the note to Annie to read.

"Well, it's just you and me, kid," said Annie, as she placed the note back on the table before heading upstairs.

Seventeen

SENSING THE FEEL

Annie bounded down the stairs after her shower feeling good about the day and her life. She had a hop to her step. As she reached the bottom of the stairs, the aroma hit her. She recognized it but couldn't quite place it. She followed the smell until she saw the pot on the kitchen table along with two bowls and an unopened bottle of Sauvignon Blanc.

"Pelican Stew," she cried out. "No way."

She spotted the note, which was written on the back of Sam's note:

Kate and Annie,
  Enjoy the stew that will bring alive all of your senses. Speaking of senses, I'll be back after you eat to take you through a short activity on this.
  Doc

Annie smiled. Good ole, Doc. She felt as if she had known him forever. She opened the wine, doled out the stew in the bowls, and waited for Kate.

"What's that wonderful smell?" asked Kate, as she ventured into the kitchen.

"Doc brought over the Pelican Stew that was in Billy's kitchen," said Annie.

"No way," said Kate. "Do you think they saw us?"

"I don't think so. Let's take it out to the deck and enjoy an evening dinner overlooking the ocean."

"Sounds good to me. Wine too!" said Kate. "Wow, I'm impressed."

Settled on the deck, Annie and Kate dug in on the stew.

"This is incredible," said Kate.

"I know. It's even better than the other night when I had it out on the beach," said Annie.

"The wine goes great with it," said Kate.

"Here's to friendship," said Annie, as she raised her glass and clinked it with Kate's.

"I'm having a great time," said Annie, in between bites of stew. "How about you?"

"Yes, it's definitely one of the most interesting vacations that I've ever been on," said Kate.

"That's an understatement," said Annie. "Thanks for playing along, Kate. I really appreciate it. I know a lot of this wasn't in the plans."

"No problem. It's been quite the adventure. What are friends for anyway?"

Kate and Annie enjoyed the ensuing silence. While they finished up their stew, they marveled at the view before them and embraced the light breeze filtering over the deck.

"Ahoy, mateys," a voice called out below. "Permission to come aboard."

"C'mon up, Doc," said Annie. "We've been expecting you."

After climbing the windy stairs, Doc plopped down in one of the chairs. He had on the customary wraparounds and wore a light jacket even though it was still quite warm.

"Thanks so much for the stew, Doc," said Annie. "It's great."

"Yes, thank you so much, Doc," said Kate.

"You're welcome. You've been playing a lot so Billy figured it's the least we could do," said Doc. "Billy suggested that I bring it over with the wine. I hope they go together. Billy knows a lot more about wine then I do."

"It's perfect," said Kate. "Would you like a glass?"

"No thanks. I'm not supposed to drink alcohol."

"But I saw you with a beer that first night," said Annie.

"Billy will drive anyone to drink," said Doc. "Moment of weakness."

Kate and Annie laughed.

"So what do you have in store for Annie tonight, Doc?" asked Kate who was catching on quickly to Doc's approach.

"Nothing too taxing, just a simple activity that you both might like playing around with," said Doc, getting warmed up. "So, Annie, in your experience over the past few days what stands out?"

"Well, I've been playing a lot. I've been exploring what's right about me. We've had some great discussions. But honestly, the thing that hit me over the head the hardest, was the realization that I don't play very much and I don't play at all with Dylan or John. Billy picked up on that. I think I invite judgment from them and so I'm not myself when I'm around them. I'm not me. That's going to be different when I get back."

Kate shook on the inside when she heard John's name.

"So how do you feel tonight compared to how you feel when you are home or at work?" Doc asked.

"I feel lighter; I feel freer. I feel more in touch with my surroundings.

"You've been smiling and laughing more," said Kate. "I've noticed that."

"Yes, yes, I believe that's true. My smile has returned and I've been paying more attention to my posture. It seems like I'm positioning my body more naturally.

"That's because you're losing weight," said Doc.

"Oh, that reminds me. The scale at the Spa said that I have lost five pounds. I didn't tell you, Kate, because I didn't want to say anything in front of Sam. I don't know how it happened but it happened."

"Are you sure the scale was right?" asked Kate.

"Yep, it's similar to the one we use at the Y," Annie replied.

"Well, that's impressive," said Kate, as she gave Annie a fist pump.

"Well, it's not really the actual weight that's important right now," Doc said, wanting to move on. "The losing weight I'm referring to is more that you are lessening the burden of responsibility and judgment that you have placed directly on your shoulders over the past many years. And we've talked a little about this, Annie, once you re-touch that clean, unspoiled spot and actively experience it, you'll more naturally want to move your body and prepare and eat foods that fuel this deep felt experience you have recaptured."

"Hey, 'fuel the feel,' that was one of the Pelican's Princ—" Kate covered her mouth, realizing that she had just put her foot in it.

"It's okay, Kate," said Doc. "Billy saw you guys leaving the shack. It's no big deal. I'm surprised you had the guts to walk in. Feel free to enter at your own risk anytime."

"I do get what you're saying, Doc," said Annie, who was more interested in processing Doc's metaphor for losing weight. "You have to lose weight to lose weight—that's the weightless way."

"Right," said Doc.

"Okay, this all makes more sense to me now," said Kate. "I kinda like it. I do have a couple of questions about those Pelican's Principles though."

"Well, hold off on those," said Doc. "Let's do this activity quickly. I call it *Sensing the Feel*. This deep felt sense that I'm talking about can sometimes be better understood through the senses. I'm just going to ask you to complete the sentence. Just take turns going first. Annie you answer the first one first."

Kate and Annie leaned forward in anticipation.

Doc started in: *"If life was a taste, I would want it to taste like…"*

"Pelican Stew," said Annie. "A slurpy after a tennis match from Seven-Eleven," Kate said, remembering her high school days.

"If life was a sound, I would want it to sound like…"

"Ocean waves." "The pop of a tennis ball coming off the racket."

If life was a smell, I would want it to smell like…"

"My YMCA." "My body after a tennis match."

"Ugh!" said Annie. "Gross."

"If life was a touch, I would want it to feel like…"

"My steering wheel when I first started to drive. "John's arms around me when we first started dating."

"Ohh, how sweet," said Kate.

"If life was a sight, I would want it to look like…"

"My kids sleeping when they were little." "My smile after we won states."

"Yes," said Annie, as she high fived with Kate. "What's the next one, Doc?"

"That's it," said Doc.

"Oh, man, that was fun. I don't want to stop," said Kate.

Kate looked at Doc. "I got this," she said.

Doc nodded.

"These are all things that Kate and I like or have liked, right?"

"And how do you know you like or liked these things?" asked Doc.

"Our senses told us," said Kate.

"Very good, Kate," said Annie.

Kate was beaming.

How easy or difficult was it for you to come up with the answers?" Doc asked.

"Super easy," said Annie.

Why?"

"Because these experiences are a natural part of who we are," said Annie.

"Even more than that," said Doc. "All of your senses make up your deep felt experiences. They help you feel life and create and grow your spot. They help you *know* what you like. Now, did you need anybody to help you complete each sentence?"

"Of course not, we are our own experts on our deep felt experience."

"That's right. Remember, Annie, what we were talking about the other day. That our body is the greatest perceptive instrument ever designed. The senses activity just reminds us that we don't need experts who know about or to rely on others to tell us how to experience our senses. We do it naturally—if you are paying attention and free from judgment."

"Wow, that was such a fun activity, Doc," said Kate. "Is this what you have been doing with Annie?"

"Mostly. It's not that much different from *The Game With No Name* or the *TurnTennis* that we played a couple of nights ago."

"It's so simple," said Kate.

"But not easy," said Annie, beating Doc to the punch.

"And it's not so easy if you aren't paying attention or if you are weighed down with responsibility and judgment," Doc reminded them.

Kate thought of Sam. That's why she resisted Doc and despised Billy. They had what she didn't, and she knew it. But Annie was so open to everything. Why? she wondered.

"Well, that's probably enough for today," said Doc. "I'm getting a little tired and you are probably getting a little tired of me."

Truth was, Doc's fingers, which he had placed in his pockets, were turning blue and his eyes were burning.

"We were thinking of taking a walk on the beach," said Annie. "Did you want to come with us? We're not getting tired of you, Doc."

"Yeah, come with us," said Kate.

"That's okay. You guys go. Enjoy it. And just keep the pot and bring it back tomorrow," Doc said, as he started down the steps of the deck to head towards the warmth of the shack.

A few minutes later, Doc watched from the shack window as Kate and Annie strolled along the beach, arm in arm. Their friendship was as natural as the senses. He thought of his few close friends scattered around the country. He thought of two in particular who had died way too young without Doc saying goodbye. He missed them all and began to cry, but no tears would come.

Day 5
Trust

Eighteen

FEEL, NOT FEELINGS

When Billy Hamilton was young he had, of course, seen the wild horses that roamed the Banks, and knew of them from informal history lessons in school. During the 1960s and 70s, it was not uncommon for these horses to appear on the beach but as the tourism grew they were relegated to areas north of White Horse Island.

One day at school, Billy had asked his 4th grade teacher where the wild horses came from. His teacher said that no one knew for sure but probably from Spanish ships that wrecked along the coast or they were brought to land by Spanish colonists.

"My dad says that pirates rode them to escape and hide from the law," one kid said.

"Highly unlikely," said the teacher.

"Well I know where the White Horses come from," Billy stated.

"You mean the wild horses right, Billy?" the teacher clarified.

"No, Ma'am, the White Horses, you know, the White Horses that play in the waves and come to shore."

Oh, the White Horses," said the teacher. "Well, that's really just a legend. There aren't really White Horses. I mean there are, but not around here, and certainly not in the ocean waves."

The other kids laughed.

"But I've seen them," said Billy.

"You have?" said one kid. "I've never seen them."

"Yeah, my grandfather told me about them. They're all white, every single one of them." The other kids in the class stopped talking. They were all ears whenever Billy talked. He was easily the smartest kid—as well as the best storyteller—in the class.

"That's just a legend, Billy," the teacher said, getting a little nervous that Billy was gearing up to take the class on another wild story ride.

"Do they really come to shore?" one kid asked Billy.

"Yeah, I've ridden them in a few times," said Billy, as the kids gathered round. "They can change into people too. That's how they escaped from Poseidon."

"Cool," said another kid. "What kinds of people do they change into?"

"Whoever you'd like them to be," said Billy. "I've played with them. So has my grandfather."

"Well, I'd like my White Horses to turn into a teacher who doesn't give us homework," a boy named Jimmy quipped.

The kids laughed.

"That's enough, Jimmy." The teacher couldn't tell if Billy seriously believed what he was saying or making it all up.

"How do you do it?" asked one kid. "How do you change them into people?"

"That's the thing," Billy said. "I don't really know. It just happens. My grandfather says that it's the magic in me. Whenever I want to play they just kind of appear."

"Okay, class, back to work," said the teacher. "That's enough storytelling for one day. Thank you, Billy."

But Billy did more than tell stories about the White Horses. He lived the legend. He called to them when it was time to play or when times got difficult. And they called to him. His grandfather had been right.

Living in a D.C. suburb that he hated, Billy started taking the bus into the city to play hoops with the black kids. He would stay all day during the summer. He liked the adventure and the challenge. At first, they made fun of him. Because of all of his practice at the Whalehead Club, Billy could shoot but that was about it. But Billy's Outer Banks upbringing made him tough and the city kids respected him for that. He watched how they played. He learned. He rebounded. He found the open man. He played tenacious defense because he didn't want to lose and sit out. All the kids wanted him on their team because they knew they wouldn't lose. Billy could be trusted to bring it every game. And then one day he actually received a pass on the wing on the fast break. Dribbling once, he lifted off the ground and glided toward the basket, long hair flying. He slammed the ball with authority into a rim with no net. The park went nuts. One kid on the other team cried out, "What the fuck was that, white boy?" Billy shrugged, grinning. A teammate said, "That was a fucking pelican, man, gliding and soaring. That was Billy fucking Pelican. He's an ugly white boy, but he's got game." And that's how William Jefferson Hamilton IV became known as Billy Pelican. Word spread fast that Billy Pelican was a damn good basketball player and by his junior year in high school Billy had scholarship offers from Division I schools up and down the East Coast.

Billy Pelican chose UVa and it was during his brief two years there that his and Annie's paths would cross, albeit briefly. But Annie gave him his life back, and now, thirty years later, Billy was trying to save hers, repaying his debt.

*U*nlike Doc, Annie's sleep was deep and restful. She woke missing John's presence, which was a feel she hadn't felt in awhile. That realization made her smile. It was already getting light, which excited her.

How do I want to feel today? she asked herself. She wasn't sure where this question came from but it was a lot better than the other one that she usually asked: What do I have to do today? She vowed to never ask herself that question again.

How do I want to feel today? Weightless, light, playful, she thought. Today she wanted to be in charge of her own play: body surfing, tennis, whatever. Two days left and she was going to make the best of it.

Annie dressed and ventured downstairs to rouse Kate. A few knocks got no reply. Quietly opening the door, Annie could see Kate under the covers, dead to the world. She didn't have the heart to wake her. Sam's door was open. It looked like she never made it back. Oh Sam, I hope you know what you're doing, Annie thought.

Out on the deserted beach, Annie placed her chair with her Cornwell novel on the seat and her towel draped over the back. She ran toward the water and dove in. An awakening! She let the water wash over her as she swam out to where her and Billy were yesterday. I'm alone. I like the feeling, she thought.

Annie spent the next hour or so practicing body surfing by herself. It had been years since she actually practiced something on her own outside of work. She tinkered with her technique. She focused on being relaxed, timing the waves. Some runs were a bust, but some she traveled all the way to the shoreline. It was exhilarating. On her last few runs, she actually tried to use her arm as a rudder and noticed that it did steer her in certain ways. On the very last run, she made it to shore and as she ended she noticed big feet standing in the water at the finish. Wiping her hair back from her eyes, she looked up to see Billy Pelican with a huge grin. He extended a hand to help her up. To her relief, Annie noticed that she didn't get all tingly anymore when Billy touched her.

"You looked practically weightless out there," said Billy.

"Thanks," said Annie.

"You've really picked it up quickly," said Billy.

"Well, I had a good teacher," said Annie, as she grabbed her towel to dry off. "What a glorious way to start the day."

"Nothing better," said Billy. "That's a big reason I moved back here."

"So you use to live here?" asked Annie.

"Well, not here exactly. Most of the locals live on the sound side. I moved to DC when I was fourteen. This place has changed a lot over the years."

"Wow, it must have been culture shock to move to DC," said Annie. "Why did you move?"

"Oh, my father and grandfather had a falling out of sorts and my father wanted his own life. He was interested in politics and law. He wanted to be where the action was."

"How did you adjust?"

"It wasn't too bad really. I found basketball. It was probably the best thing for me because I discovered I loved competition. I would have never gotten a basketball scholarship to UVa if I had gone to high school around here."

"You must have been at UVa a little before me," said Annie. "I started fall of 81."

"Yeah, I was only there two years and then transferred during summer of 81."

"Oh, man, I just missed you," Annie said.

"Fast forward and here we are," said Billy.

Annie got the sense that Billy wanted to tell her something. This time she waited out the silence but nothing. Annie wanted to change the subject but couldn't think of anything to say.

"So I have today and tomorrow to finish up my White Horse Island weightless program," she finally blurted out. "I'm a little nervous about going back and holding on to what I've done here."

"What do you think you've done?" asked Billy.

"Well, I know I've touched and felt my spot. I feel more like me than ever before. I feel lighter. I've actually lost weight. Play and you and Doc brought me back to life, and for that I am forever grateful. But I just keep wondering if it's me or this place? What will happen when I'm home, when I'm at work?"

"Haven't heard that one before," Billy said, covering up because he knew he was going to get hit.

Annie swished the towel at him. "But seriously how do people hold on to what's right about them when they discover it in a place like this? What if their environment isn't a good fit for what they've discovered?"

"The simple answer is that you have to trust it," Billy said. "And I know it will be difficult, you will hit obstacles, but you can do this."

"Are you trying to build up my confidence?" Annie asked.

"Confidence is overrated. I'm talking more about trusting what you have felt here. And as far as the environment goes, I assume you're not going to quit your job or get a divorce?"

"No, I like my job overall and I do love John."

"Okay, so what has been weighing you down in these areas? How can you bring yourself into these experiences at work and at home?"

"I'm not sure what you mean." Said Annie.

"Well, Doc told me that one of your favorite things to do at work is to hang out with or interact with some of your older members. Why?"

"I don't know. They're so vibrant and alive. They're funny."

"They don't judge you, do they?"

"No, they accept me for who I am. They just like me and I like them."

"So why wouldn't you make a point to work out with them or hang out with them on a more regular basis? That's why you got into Y work in the first place, isn't it?"

"I don't know, I always find work to do—"

"Which weighs you down, which evokes negative feelings, which makes you turn to comfort food to quiet the feelings instead of taking the time to feel the food that would inform your energy, and the gaining weight cycle continues."

"Yes, that's exactly right. Is that what you meant by "feel, not feelings" as one of your Pelican's Principles?"

"Yes, Doc told me that you and Kate visited my humble abode. I hope it wasn't too scary."

Annie laughed out loud.

Billy continued: "Feelings are just immediate reactions to experiences. For the most part, they aren't very useful. The whole emotional intelligence thing doesn't tell the whole story. That's why constant judgment is so dangerous because it evokes negative feelings, which typically make us feel bad, which weighs us down even more. If you don't know how you want to feel, when you go out into the world each day in that way it's very easy to invite judgment and act according to the resultant feelings. Judgment and feelings go hand in hand. But now you are clearer on how you want to feel. You have to trust that you know your feel and what brings it alive because people will tell you that you don't, shit will happen. People will want to drag you back into their world of judgment and feelings. Trust helps you rise above."

"Kind of like the swing discussion we had the other night about like versus want."

"Yes, exactly, when the world pulls you back down, how do you swing back up again to experience that beautiful feel at the top of the swing—when the world stands still for you. Just a simple moment working out with people you respect and admire and accepting you for who you are can provide enough informed energy to give you a push back up."

"Fuel the feel," Annie said.

"Man, what did you do, memorize all of the principles?"

"Most of them. I think it's helped that I've been experiencing most of them. I do want to ask about the goals principle."

"You should probably talk with Doc about that one. He put that one in there. I don't give a shit about goals…well, I should get my surfing in before the non Pelicans start strutting around on the beach. What are you going to do today?"

"Not too many plans—lay out, play some tennis, maybe create my own *Game With No Name.*

"Cool…hey, I was thinking that maybe we could have a big clambake tomorrow night on the beach to give you an appropriate send off."

"That sounds wonderful. Will you need any help?"

"I'll let you know," Billy said, as he ran into the water and disappeared into the White Horses.

Annie sat in the chair and watched Billy for a while, which was more interesting than the book. His movements seemed so pure, like he was dancing with the water. For a brief moment, it looked to Annie like Billy was one of the White Horses.

Nineteen

SAVING SAM

Annie had just finished her breakfast of fruit and yogurt and was pondering what to do next when Sam walked in with Harry.

"Hi Lil Orphan Annie," said Sam.

"Hi Sam Suntan," said Annie. "Where have you been or should I even ask?"

"We've been enjoying each other's company," said Sam, holding on to Harry's arm. Harry smiled. He actually seemed to be enjoying hanging out with Sam. The sex last night was even better than he thought it would be.

"Where's Kate because I have a big surprise?" said Sam.

"I'm not sure. She wasn't here when I got back from body surfing. I've tried her cell but no answer. Don't tell me you two are engaged or something crazy like that?"

"No, silly, but Harry is good friends with the guy in charge of hang gliding over at Jockey's Ridge, you know, where we were a couple of days ago. Well, we ran into him at breakfast this morning and he's willing to give us a free lesson. But we have to be there in like 30 minutes. He's got an opening where no one's scheduled for ten o'clock.

"Hang gliding?" asked Annie.

"It's pretty low key," said Harry. "They have a beginner's hill and they pretty much hold on to you the whole time. It's idiot proof. I think you get five flights. The feeling of flying is pretty cool. I highly recommend it."

"So I'm an idiot?" Annie teased.

"Well…no…of course not," said Harry.

"I'm kidding, Harry," said Annie. "It sounds like fun. But what about Kate?"

"Leave her a note," said Sam. "Tell her where we are. She can always drive the rental to join us if she gets the note in time."

"Okay. But you write the note. I'm going up to change. I'll be quick."

While Annie did a quick change, she marveled at her new-found sense of adventure. A few days ago she would have hemmed and hawed and come up with some excuse not to go. Her mind floated back to the time when she and her brother pretended to be Superwoman and Superman and jumped off the garage with capes they had worn as part of their Halloween costumes. She made it safely but her brother broke his ankle and they were both grounded for a month. Of course, her brother couldn't do anything anyway so it was much tougher on Annie. As the older one, she was assigned to "take care" of her brother, which was mental torture, as he demanded services of her similar to that of a hotel concierge.

Annie bounded down the stairs. "Let's go," she exclaimed. As they were pulling out in Harry's Jeep, Doc pulled up on Billy's bike, fresh from a morning ride.

"Hi, Doc," said Annie.

"Where you guys going?" Doc asked with a bit of trepidation, feeling skeptical of anything that might involve Sam. He did not want Sam ruining the internal process that Annie had begun with touch, feel, play, and know. He knew that trusting the process was an essential element to ultimately creating and experiencing a eudaimonic life, full of purpose and meaning.

"We're heading for hang gliding at Jockey's Ridge," said Harry. "Come with us, Doc. Should be fun. Hop in." Sam winced at the thought of Doc joining them.

"Yeah, c'mon, Doc," said Annie.

"Yeah, please join us," said Sam, sarcastically.

Heights, ugh! thought Doc, remembering his recent dunes debacle. But he knew he had no choice. He couldn't leave Annie alone with Sam, not now. "Am I okay with what I have on?" Doc asked, referring to his cycling attire.

"Sure," said Harry.

Doc rested Billy's bike and helmet on the side of the drive, jumped in the back with Annie, and the merry group zoomed off to Jockey's Ridge. Doc hung on for dear life as Harry made like Jeff Gordon driving in the Brickyard 400.

Pulling in to the Park's parking lot, Annie laughed at Doc as they got out of the Jeep.

"What?" asked Doc.

"Your hair. You look like Woody Woodpecker," said Annie.

Harry and Sam couldn't help but laugh as well.

"He kind of acts like a little pecker too," said Sam.

"SAM," said Harry and Annie.

Doc couldn't think of an appropriate comeback so he had to let it go. He couldn't call Sam an ignorant slut or anything derogatory in front of Harry as he had saved their ass this week.

At the training center, they met Dutch, Harry's friend, and the hang gliding guru. Dutch was ripped, tan, and looked like a former football player who could still maul a quarterback. He was also overly enthusiastic about the beauty of hang gliding and was a man in constant motion as he took Sam, Annie, and Doc through about 45 minutes of training, which included a video explaining correct technique and safety guidelines.

Dutch assured them of the safety of the hang gliding experience as he pushed the "Waiver and Release of Liability" in front of them to sign.

It was at that point that Doc dropped out of the active participant pool. Although the Waiver wasn't directly responsible for his decision, phrases such as "…is a physically demanding and inherently dangerous sport" or "I understand I may suffer a broken limb, paralysis or fatal injury while participating in the sport of Flying" didn't help to motivate him to participate. He didn't see hang gliding as a sport and the only place he wanted to suffer was at Sunday mass.

As they hiked their way over to the beginner dunes, Dutch explained that the day's Southeast wind would mean that the gliders would take off towards the ocean rather than the sound. "The light breeze is perfect for flying," said Dutch. "Too much wind and the gliders can be hard to control."

The group gave Doc a hard time about his decision but he stuck to it. He was getting a weird vibe and felt that his place was to stand near the landing area to watch and cheer.

Doc looked on as Dutch and Harry carried the gliders up to the top of the take off hill. He couldn't help but watch Sam from behind as well. When they reached the top, he watched Dutch hook up the women's harnesses to each glider. Annie and Sam then took turns learning how to fly. Annie's first attempt ended about halfway down the hill with a face plant in the sand. Both Harry and Dutch ran alongside holding some kind of safety cord, helping to balance the wings. Annie's next couple of flights were much better, although she didn't quite reach Doc.

On Sam's third attempt, Harry and Dutch let go of the safety cords, and she actually reached Doc. He had to move out of the way to avoid getting bowled over. She made a perfect landing—upright and standing.

Doc was impressed. It was obvious Sam was a natural. "Good one, Sam," said Doc.

"Thanks, Woody," said Sam, laughing.

Doc turned away to control his emotions, and it was then that he noticed how close they were to the ocean—just a long home run away from Highway 158 and Highway 12, the beach homes, the beach, and then the ocean. Doc tried to estimate the distance to the ocean, about 600 to 800 yards, he thought. About two laps around the track, Doc thought, thinking back to his days when he did speed work in preparation for road races. He loved speed work and got lost in his reminiscing.

It was a good thing Doc turned around when he did because he could see Sam bearing down on him. He quickly sidestepped her as she landed a few yards behind where he had been just standing.

"Look lively, Woody," Sam teased. "You never know when a hot chick might be coming after you."

"Thanks for the warning," said Doc, as Harry and Dutch caught up and unhooked Sam from the glider. "I'll be on the lookout for one."

Dutch and Harry, raving about Sam's skill, started carrying the glider back leaving Sam and Doc out of ear shot.

"Watch this last one, Doc. I'm going to take off from the higher dunes and go for a long ride."

Doc's antennae went up. He couldn't help himself. "Well, just be careful, Sam."

"Oh, Doc, I didn't know you cared. Don't worry, I know what I'm doing."

How many times had Doc heard the phrase "don't worry, I know what I'm doing." It usually signaled overconfidence and performance disaster. How many conversations had he and Billy had about the difference between trust and confidence? Billy had learned from the best of the best that confidence was fleeting, artificial, overrated. Trust was something you built from touch and feel and play. Sam had no business being confident about what Doc thought was a potentially dangerous activity.

Doc watched as the trio hiked up the eighty foot dunes that they had rolled down the other day. Annie trailed behind, probably wanting to support Sam's final run.

What happened in the next few minutes will forever be a blur in Doc's memory. Later, Dutch would say that Sam must have hit a rare thermal that just carried her up, up, and away.

Sam started running before Dutch and Harry could grab the safety cords. Doc watched in horror as Sam, just a few seconds after lift off, flew much higher than he knew she should have. She must have panicked because instead of beginning a descent to land on the sand, she was ascending. Doc watched as Harry and Dutch ran down the dunes, knowing there was big trouble brewing. Dutch was yelling something up to Sam that Doc couldn't make out.

As Sam was getting closer to the landing area, Doc realized that she was flying much too fast and still too high. She'll never make it, Doc thought. Doc had never been in an emergency situation where he had to act and act quickly. He always felt it odd that in the fifty plus years of his life there had never been a day when his life or someone else's was directly on the line—that he or someone else he knew might face imminent death. Today was that day. The moment was now. It just so happened that it was Sam Pennington's life that was on the line.

"DOC, HELP," Sam cried out from above.

"SAM, YOU'VE GOT TO MAKE THE BEACH. LAND IT ON THE BEACH," Doc yelled upwards while pointing to the ocean. "I'LL TRY TO CATCH UP TO YOU."

"HURRY, DOC."

Doc looked back. He saw Dutch and Harry, already winded; they would never make it. Annie was trailing far back.

"CALL 911," yelled Doc, as he threw his phone to them.

It was up to Doc.

He turned and started running in the sand, looking up to see where Sam was heading.

Doc bounded through the prickly sea grass, saw an opening, and reached Highway 158. All senses were alive as he gauged traffic and speed and looked left and right for any sign of a road heading toward the beach. Spotting a traffic light to his right, he turned in that direction. With no traffic, he ran down the center of Highway 158 and then left on to a road traveling east-west. He gave a quick look skyward and saw that Sam was circling down a bit. Turning left on to the side road, he picked up speed. Bell lap, he told himself. In what seemed like forever, he finally reached Highway 12 and had to dodge a car heading south. He bolted across the highway, saw an opening in between two beach houses, and scampered through. As he neared the opening to the beach, he looked up in time to see Sam's glider veer sharply to the left and then take a nose dive. He heard someone yell "Oh my God" from one of the houses. Doc saw the glider, out of control, crash into the water about 200 yards north. He kicked off his shoes and sunglasses and looked around for help. The beach was empty. "Fuck," he muttered. He feared the worst, and began an all out sprint, adrenaline taking over, his body flying over the sand. As he reached the water, it appeared that Sam was farther out than he had thought. He ran into the waves as far as he could and then dove in, his lungs burning for oxygen. Doc was no swimmer but he trudged through the ocean waves as best he could, taking in a lot of water.

Finally, Doc reached Sam, who was floating face down, blood trickling down the side of her head. Unconscious. Holding on to the glider's steering bar with one hand, Doc reached up to unhook Sam's harness. He was thankful he went through the training, as he knew how to unlock the caribineer. He unsnapped Sam's helmet strap, gently pulled the helmet off her head, and flung it into the ocean.

Mustering up his strength from somewhere deep inside, he rolled Sam over on her back, trying to keep her head above water with his left arm underneath her neck. Then he began to push his right arm through the water to head towards shore. He took a deep breath just before his head submerged. He was moving but ever so slowly. Coming up for air, he rotated to the left and was able to get his right arm under Sam's left armpit. He turned towards shore and using a scissors kick made better progress. Just as he was about to go under from the weight, his feet touched bottom. Doc stood up, quickly grabbed Sam under the arms, and dragged her through the water.

Doc heard sirens, which gave him hope. As he reached shore, he gasped for breath and placed Sam softly on the sand. He took a moment to jog his memory from the CPR class that his colleague at the university had forced him to attend with her last summer. "You never know," she had said. "ABC," Doc said to himself. "Airways, Breathing, Circulation."

He checked the airway for blockages with his fingers. He leaned over Sam's face to check for breathing. Nothing. He tilted Sam's head back, pinched her nose, covered her mouth with his, and pumped two quick breaths of air into her lungs. He looked to see if her chest moved. Nothing. He tried the rescue breaths again. Nothing. He checked her carotid artery for a pulse. Nothing. Doc began the chest compressions and followed up with the rescue breaths. Nothing. He did it again. He saw Sam's chest rise, her beautiful chest. Then he heard her cough.

Two EMTs arrived. "She's breathing," Doc said, as he collapsed to the sand under the weight of fatigue and exhaustion. The EMTs stabilized her head and gently placed her on the stretcher. "Nice job," said one of the EMTs to Doc. "We're taking her to the Outer Banks Medical Center ER just down the road. Her vitals look good. I think she'll be all right."

"What about the blood?" Doc asked.

"Looks like just a scratch. She doesn't seem to have any broken bones or anything."

Harry, Dutch, and Annie arrived on the scene in Harry's beach-friendly Jeep. Doc gave a thumbs up as they rushed over.

Before the EMTs placed Sam in the ambulance, she motioned with her hand for Doc to come over.

"I saw the White Horses, Doc," she whispered. "I saw them just before I crashed."

Harry, Annie, and Doc spent most of the afternoon in the ER waiting room. The ER doc talked with them a few times about how great Sam was doing. As a precaution, he wanted to admit Sam overnight for observation, and if everything went smoothly, she could be released the following morning. Kate joined them at the hospital as well once she got word, and brought Doc a change of clothes that Billy gave her. Once Sam was in her hospital room, they were allowed to visit.

Annie and Kate gave Sam hugs as did Harry.

"C'mon over here, Doc," Sam said, as she raised her arms for a hug.

Doc reluctantly allowed Sam to hug him. "Thank you, Doc. You saved my life."

"Ah, no big deal," said Doc.

"You should have seen Doc running, Sam," said Harry. "I couldn't keep up."

"He was a beast," said Annie.

"How did you get me out of the water, Doc?" asked Sam. "The last thing I remember is crashing."

"Well, I just unstrapped you from the glider and pulled you to shore. Good thing you're light. Maybe the White Horses helped," Doc said with a wink.

"Maybe," said Sam, smiling. "Hey, would you guys mind, I want to talk with Annie privately."

When the others left the room, Annie came over and sat on the edge of Sam's bed. "What's up?" she asked.

"I want to apologize for my behavior the past few days," said Sam. She reached for Annie's hand.

"It's okay," said Annie. "You probably felt left out of some of things I've been doing with Doc and Billy. It hasn't been the normal vacation."

"I was envious of all of the attention you were getting. I should have been more supportive. I haven't always been a good friend over the years."

"Yes, you have. We're fine. You should just get some rest."

"Thanks, Annie. I do have something else I need to tell you."

"What's that?

Sam took a deep breath. "Well, when we were in college I had sex with John…but it was before you met him."

"I know," said Annie.

"You know?" asked Sam.

"Yes, John told me shortly after we started dating."

"He did?"

"Yep. We've always been very honest with each other. Thanks for sending him my way way back when."

"Uh…so…we're good then?" asked Sam.

"Unless you've got any other secrets to reveal," said Annie.

"Well, I do but none that involve you. I think that's about it," said Sam, squeezing Annie's hand. "I love you Lil Orphan Annie."

"I love you Sam Suntan. Now get some rest."

Harry stayed most of the evening with Sam. He told her his life story and as Sam drifted off to sleep he told her that he loved her.

Twenty

GOALS COME LATER, IF AT ALL

Later that day, Kate drove Annie and Doc from the hospital back to White Horse Island. As they neared the rental house, Annie spotted *White Horse Fish Company*, a little hole-in-the-wall, roadside eatery and told Kate to pull over.

"I say this is our dinner tonight kids," said Annie.

"Looks good to me," said Doc, who had been fighting nodding off in the back seat. He hadn't ever had an experience like today and it had sapped most of his energy.

"Let's go see what they have," said Kate.

"Do you guys want to take it home or do you want to eat it here?" asked Annie, as she got out of the car.

"I vote for home," said Kate.

"Me too," said Doc.

There wasn't much to the place. It reminded Annie of Billy's shack. Picnic tables and benches were outside for those that wanted to eat their catch on the premises. Walking inside, Annie was hit with the smell of fish. A small TV was playing behind the register. A gregarious, younger woman greeted them and Annie immediately thought of the difference between her greeting and that of the woman at the Spa. She knew this place would have great seafood.

"What can I get you folks?" the woman asked.

"Well, we're interested in take out," said Annie. "Do you have that?"

"Sure," said the woman, handing Annie the take out menu. "If you're all together, you might want to get one of our steamer combos. It will take a bit to prepare but well worth the wait."

"Okay," said Annie, as she shared the menu with Doc and Kate. They all agreed that the Seafarer Combo was perfect and they ordered a quart of clam chowder, Doc's favorite, on the side.

After placing their order, they walked outside and sat at one of the picnic tables.

"Just so you guys know," said Annie "this dinner is on me."

Doc was too tired to argue. Kate put up a little resistance but in the end succumbed to Annie's persistence.

They reviewed the day's events and Annie was still gushing about Doc's heroic dash to save Sam, while thinking about her own rescue mission thirty years ago. It was still fuzzy to Doc, even when he was talking to the TV and newspaper reporters at the hospital; it seemed like a surreal event, like it never happened. He was proud of himself for being prepared and acting quickly, but he felt it was destiny that he happened to be wearing his running shoes and standing in that very spot—the right moment at the right time. There wasn't much else he could do but run after Sam, like his behavior really wasn't under his control.

"I'm kind of sorry I missed all the excitement," said Kate.

"Yea, where were you this morning?" asked Sam.

"Well, no one was at the house when I woke up so I walked over to the Spa. They had an opening so I actually had a session with Meg, the well-ness coach.

Suddenly Doc wasn't tired anymore. His antennae were up.

"You did?" asked Annie.

"Yep, sure did," said Kate.

"How was it?" asked Annie, as she saw Doc grimace.

"Well, better than I thought. We focused on what I was interested in doing and how I was going to get there. She really listened. We talked about self-efficacy, or confidence, and goals, especially relating to my desire to be more physically active."

"That sounds interesting," said Annie.

"Meg said that the most important element in changing behavior is to set goals," Kate said.

Doc put his head in his hands and rubbed his temples. How many times did had he read that line in the health coaching manuals. "Were they smart goals?" asked Doc.

"Yes, smart goals," said Kate. "That's right, Doc, smart goals. Smart is an acronym for something. I can't quite remember…"

"…S is for specific, M is measurable, A is action-based, R is realistic, and T is for time-line. S…M…A…R…T." Doc recited the letters in a monotone, rhythmic manner.

"Yes, Meg said that all goals should have those elements," Kate said.

"What's the matter, Doc, you aren't too keen on goals?" Annie asked, based on seeing his body language.

"We probably don't have the time to get into it now," said Doc, "and I don't think you really want to hear my version anyway, do you?"

"YES WE DO," Kate and Sam said in unison.

"It's one of the questions I've been wanting to ask ever since I saw it listed on *Pelican's Principles*: Goals come later, if at all," said Kate.

Doc wasn't used to adults actually being interested in what he had to say lately. Most of his faculty colleagues certainly weren't interested in anything that might muddy their teaching waters. He needed a new circle of friends beyond his wife, his kids, and college students, who were a captive audience and had no choice but to listen.

"Well, I've examined goals from every angle," Doc started in. "I've read the theories and the research. I've listened in on coaching sessions. And I've talked to Billy for hours on end about this. My basic conclusion is that when it comes to health and well-being, goals the way they are typically set and used are anything but smart. They are D…U…M…B. Dumb."

Hearing no resistance, Doc continued: "When I first started out conceptualizing the Personal Exercise Program, I included goals as a means for overcoming obstacles to physical activity—"

"Wait a second, are you talking about the *Personal Exercise Program* for the YMCA? Are you talking about PEP?" Annie asked, as she jumped out of her picnic bench.

"Yes," said Doc.

"Oh…my…God," said Annie.

"What, what?" asked Kate.

"Doc is the guy who helped create this program, PEP, that's been around the Y for years. I've used it in my Y. I can't believe this. Now I remember. Doc, I heard you speak at this national Y conference way back when. I was sitting way in the back but I was on board from day one. I can't believe I didn't recognize you. Must be the sunglasses. Why didn't you say something?"

"That was a lifetime ago," Doc said. "I've gone through many lives based on some philosophical shifts in how I approach physical activity, health, and well-being. And my appearance is a little different from back then."

"But I knew there was something familiar about you. I can't believe it," said Annie. "I just can't believe that the PEP guy is on my case."

Annie reached out her hand: "Hello, I'm Annie Jackson, executive director of the Charlottesville YMCA."

Doc shook Annie's hand: "I'm Jack Kozikowski, case worker. My friends call me, Doc or Doctor K, mostly because it's easier than trying to say and spell my last name."

"Okay, okay," said Kate. "I'm glad you two have re-discovered each other. But what about goals, Doc? What about goals?"

"Most people who set goals pertaining to their health and well-being don't ever attain them and even for the minority of folks who do, achieving goals like the ones you are talking about, Kate, leave a hollow feeling. They don't really enhance one's inner world. They don't create a lot of meaning for the people who achieve them."

"But why, why wouldn't goals work? I mean if I set a goal of losing ten pounds in three months, I would be ecstatic if I made it," Kate argued.

"I got this, Doc," said Annie. "Because the goal probably isn't connected to the spot, Kate. You didn't spend enough time on touch, feel, play. So you can't really know or trust that what you are doing is going to lead to something you can create for yourself that will last, that will have meaning to you."

Thank the Lord for the Annie Jacksons of the world, thought Doc. He immediately felt lighter. "I think that is spot on," said Doc. "Pun intended. You just end up setting a goal, whether it is an action goal or an outcome goal, that won't enhance the meaning of the experience. It's not something you can trust or that builds trust within yourself."

Doc paused to see if they wanted him to continue. Annie and Kate both gave him the nod.

"Many people who set goals don't know why they are setting them. People think that they will feel a certain way when they reach or achieve the goal. They try to motivate themselves to do a behavior or perform certain acts based on the idea that they will feel real good when the goal is achieved. But goals—even achieving goals—do little to enrich one's life unless they are intimately connected to a powerful underlying purpose that emanates from within—the spot. Researchers call them self-concordant goals but the name isn't all that important. That's why one of *Pelican's Principles* is *goals come later, if at all.* Goals will only be optimal when individuals have done the internal work necessary and connect those goals to a way of being that a person can really feel."

"But it sounded so…so motivating when Meg was discussing goals with me," Kate said.

"I don't want to dismiss, Meg," said Doc, "but most wellness coaches seem motivating when you are talking with them. But what happens after that? We didn't mention goals once to Annie this week."

"That's right, you didn't," said Annie. "And, hey, I lost five pounds. Weight loss without really trying. The weightless way!"

"Well, that is curious," said Kate. "Meg said I should do scale weighing so that I could measure progress. I walked down to the women's locker room when we were finished and weighed myself. Guess what?"

"What?" asked Annie.

Doc prepared himself.

"I've lost five pounds since I've been here too?" said Kate, excitedly.

"Wow, that's great," said Annie, who kicked Doc underneath the picnic table.

"Oh…yeah, that's great, Kate," said Doc, not sure if he should come clean or not.

"As I was walking back to the house," explained Kate, "it dawned on me that if I can lose five pounds by just hanging around Annie, what do I need coaching and goals for. I'll just have what she's having at White Horse Island."

"*When Harry met Sally*, 1989," said Annie.

"Very good," said Kate, turning to Doc. "Does any of this make any sense, Doc? Losing weight without really trying?"

Doc hesitated. He was hoping the take out would have been ready by now.

"Well, it's not as easy as it seems," Doc started in slowly. "I mean Annie has been doing a lot of work this week, it's just a different kind of work. We set it up so she could immerse herself in the experience of being herself and then she started doing that on her own."

"Yes, yes, I get all that," Kate said. "But why would I lose weight too?"

"Well…there is this thing called social contagion that a Harvard researcher has been working on that could explain your weight loss.

"Social what?" asked Annie.

"Social contagion," Doc repeated, "you know, like an epidemic or infection that spreads rapidly.

"Interesting," said Kate. "Explain."

Doc was grasping at straws. He knew there was something to this science but he didn't want to sound like a bullshitting expert.

"Well, this guy's research basically shows that there is a powerful connection between social networks and health. In one study he found that people who are surrounded by many happy people central to their social network are more likely to be happier in the future. People who hang around overweight people are more likely to be overweight in the future, and so on. The punch line, at least for me, is that your immediate social network is vital to your health and well-being. So why couldn't it be that your best friend, Kate, was positively infected by your experience here at White Horse Island? Social contagion. Annie loses weight to lose weight and so does Kate."

Doc stopped, realizing that he came up with a rhythmic phrase. Kate and Annie fist-bumped. "Yeah, why not," said Kate.

"Number 47" a voice came out over the outside speakers.

"That's us," said Annie, looking at her piece of paper. They walked inside together and Doc was happy for the diversion. He wasn't sure if he really believed what he just said or if he just pulled it out of his ass to hide the truth about the weight scale.

At the register, the customer-friendly woman was ringing them up and then did a double take as she looked up at her three customers.

"AHHHHHHH," the woman screamed, making Doc jump almost out of his shoes. "You're the guy," she said, pointing at Doc. "You were just on TV, on the news. You saved that runaway hang glider who crashed in the sea today."

Doc blushed. Annie and Kate smiled, patting Doc on the back. "You're famous, Doc," said Kate. "You're a hero," said Annie.

Doc smiled. It was a long time since he'd been regionally famous.

"I tell you what," said the woman, "dinner is on the *White Horse Fish Company* tonight. I can't make a hero and his entourage pay for the greatest tasting steamer combo on the Banks."

"THANK YOU," they all said in unison.

"We gratefully accept your hospitality," said Annie, as Kate and Doc turned to go. But just before Annie's right hand reached the bag full of food, the woman gently grabbed her right wrist and whispered, "Good luck with your case, honey."

Twenty-One

BACK TO THE SPA

Doc, Kate, and Annie enjoyed sharing the shrimp, clams, crawfish, and lobster as part of the Seafarer Combo. But Doc's favorite was still the clam chowder. Not much was said as they savored every morsel.

Doc was getting tired. His body wasn't used to the stress it had experienced in today's rescue. But Annie and Kate were still fired up from the day's events and suggested a walk to maybe get a peek of the sunset on the sound side.

This time Doc agreed. A short walk and then early to bed to be refreshed for Annie's last day felt right. After cleanup, they started out on the path heading towards the Spa. The sound of the water, the feel of the breeze, and the engaging conversation made Doc feel good about the way things had gone this week. He had made a few mistakes, but, overall, he felt he had been a good right hand man to carry out Billy's first, official life detective case. He still wasn't sure how and why the rescue of Sam had occurred. He was so deep in thought that he didn't notice the woman cyclist heading toward them. As she neared Doc, she slowed and took a long, hard look, almost knocking Doc over.

"HEY," shouted Doc as he scrambled to avoid contact.

"Sorry," said the cyclist, who stopped just short to take a closer look.

"You're the guy," she said in a way that didn't sound like how you would greet the day's hero.

"What guy?" asked Doc, who recognized the woman and knew that he could be in hot shit. Stay cool, Doc told himself.

"Sorry, but do we know you?" asked Annie, who was perturbed that their pleasant walk had been interrupted. She didn't yet recognize the woman as the blonde receptionist from the Spa.

"Yes, you do," the blonde said as she took off her helmet. "You're that crazy woman who ran out of the Spa yesterday."

"Oh, you're the receptionist," said Annie. "I'm sorry about yesterday, I just lost control of myself."

"No problem. But just a point of correction, I'm called a *greeter*, not a receptionist.

"Sorry," Annie said. "But how do you know Doc?" pointing at Doc.

"Well *Doc* here delivered a defective weight scale to us yesterday," the woman said. "Where's your tall friend, you know, the handsome one with that gorgeous silver hair. Man, I could look at him all day."

Annie and Kate looked at each other, *Harry*?

Doc was busted and to make matters worse, he had brain fog. His brain couldn't conjure up any good excuse or any defense other than denial.

"I don't know what you're talking about," said Doc.

"It's no big deal," said the woman. "We replaced it with a new scale. The one you gave us was registering five pounds under weight and we couldn't fix it."

Wow, Ian and Mac must have performed admirably in making that scale, thought Doc. "That's impossible," said Doc. "You must have me mistaken for someone else. I didn't deliver any scale to the Spa. I'm just visiting White Horse for the week."

"Okay, if you say so but if you run into your friend, let him know that I'm available," the woman said, as she pedaled off.

Doc waved, trying to prolong the inevitable conversation with Kate and Annie.

"Doc, I can't believe you would pull such an underhanded trick," said Annie, breaking the uncomfortable silence.

"How could you," said Kate. "Annie and I believed we really lost five pounds."

"I don't know what that woman is talking about," said Doc, turning to face the two women. "I swear I did not deliver a scale to the Spa yesterday." Doc's fatigue was making him incoherent, making his lie sound presidential.

"Oh, so if we walked over there right now, you're telling us that we would weigh the same as yesterday," said Katie.

"Well…not necessarily. The Spa's scale may have been off but I'm telling you I did not deliver that scale."

"I'd like to believe you," said Annie.

"Let's go," said Kate.

"Where?" said Annie.

"To the Spa," Kate said. "Now, I'm curious as to what I really weigh."

"Are they open?" asked Annie.

"I think till eight," Doc said.

"C'mon, Doc, you're coming with us," said Annie, pulling him by the arm. Doc's fatigue was overwhelming now. He could barely move. But he didn't have much choice. Thelma and Louise were on a mission. Doc felt like dead man walking.

As they entered the Spa, Doc slumped in one of the rattan chairs in the foyer to wait for the women to return with the weight report. Doc's tired brain tried to think of a way out of the mess he had created. He had simply tried to keep Annie away from the Spa, to keep her mind and body focused on the process of losing weight. He forced himself to stay awake by softly singing Margaritaville.

A few minutes later, Doc saw the two friends walking down the hall, heading towards him. He braced to tell the truth and hope for the best. But as they got closer, he noticed Kate and Annie were smiling and laughing.

"Well, Doc, guess what?" asked Annie.

"I'm too tired to guess," said Doc.

"We both were the same weight as yesterday," Kate gushed. "Can you believe it?"

"We've both lost five pounds," said Annie. "Now, you're sure you had nothing to do with this?"

"Scout's honor," croaked Doc, whose voice was getting hoarse from the dry mouth. "Can we go home now?"

On the walk back to the shack, Doc half listened as Annie and Kate discussed how they had lost the weight in such a short amount of time. They were bubbly and giddy, like school girls. Doc said his goodbyes as they neared the shack and he could still hear the two women laughing as he entered the shack, greeted by Obi, the ball-fetching wonder.

As his head hit the pillow, Doc was dizzy from trying to figure out how the new scale registered the same weight for Annie and Kate as Ian and Mac's homemade one. He still didn't fully appreciate the magic of the White Horses and White Horse Island. Just before he fell asleep, he reminded himself to ask Billy about it in the morning. And that night, for the first night since being diagnosed with Sjogren's Syndrome, Doc slept straight through until the sun rose over the water, flashing a wondrous beam of magical light into his tiny bedroom window.

Day 6
Create

Twenty-Two

The Good Samaritan

William Jefferson Hamilton IV's life changing moment occurred on June 13, 1981. Earlier that Saturday, the head coach of UVa's men's basketball team had notified Billy that he was revoking his scholarship due to "academic inadequacies" and an inability to meet "participation expectations." Billy spent most of the afternoon and evening drinking and smoking away his sorrow in his one-bedroom apartment, wondering how for two years of his life he had failed both on the court and in the classroom. Now the Pelican was officially grounded.

Later that night, his mind full of booze and pot and numb from his downward spiral as both a student and a former basketball star, Billy grabbed the car keys and went for a joyless, solo ride. Thoughts of suicide ran through his mind as he raced through the country roads on the outskirts of Charlottesville.

The young woman driving home from a friend's graduation party had just graduated from Charlottesville High School that evening. She had been attending a party at her classmate's country estate. The young woman also had too much to drink and had just experimented with pot for the first time with some of her celebrating classmates. The group had snuck out to the barn unbeknownst to the friend's parents, rolled a few joints, and got high. As it got later and later, her boyfriend got more and more obnoxious, and she decided to leave for home without him. As Billy headed north to nowhere on Pebble Creek Road, the woman headed south towards town on Pebble Creek Road. Both drivers approached dead man's curve out of control with speeds unsuitable for the dramatic bend in the road. As the woman went into the turn, she saw the oncoming lights and somehow swerved to avoid contact. She skidded but miraculously regained control of the car and stopped. Now fully awake, she looked in her rearview mirror in time to see the other car flipping over and crashing on the passenger side into a tree that safeguarded entry to the creek. She watched in horror as the front of the upside-down car burst into flames, lighting up the night.

The woman dashed out of her car, grabbed the quilt from the back seat that had been used for spontaneous love rendezvouses with her boyfriend, and ran towards the burning vehicle.

"HELLO," she yelled, as she reached the car.

"Help me," the young man cried out. "I can't move. I think my leg is broken."

The fire had not yet reached the man but it soon would.

She put the quilt over her hand and tried to open the door. No luck.

"The door won't open," she said frantically. "It's jammed."

"You've got to open it. Please hurry, the fire."

The woman tried again, pulling harder. The door creaked and then opened with a force that almost knocked her over. The huge man was not wearing his seat belt. The heat was unbearable.

"Can you move at all?" asked the woman.

"I'll try," the man replied. "Try to get your hands under my shoulders and pull."

The woman followed orders and as she pulled, the man screamed in pain as he tried to push his legs against the hood for leverage. He moved—slightly. Motivated by hope, the woman moved in further with her hands under his armpits and pulled again. Again, a scream, but the man was about halfway out of the car. She pulled one more time and he was out.

"Can you get up?" the woman asked. "We need to get away from the car. I don't think I'm strong enough to drag you."

"I'll try," the man said.

The woman got in behind him and tried to raise up what seemed to her a giant of a man. He rose ever so slowly and she moved in so she could get underneath his right arm. He hopped away on his good leg as the young woman held the brunt of his weight with her small, but strong, frame.

As they reached the side of the road, the man collapsed to the ground as the car exploded.

"Oh my God!" the young woman exclaimed, turning to see the car completely engulfed in flames.

The woman covered the man with the quilt. He was between that gray area of conscious and unconscious.

"What's your name?" Billy asked in a whisper of a voice.

"Annie," she said.

"Annie the Angel," Billy said.

"What's your name?" Annie asked, but Billy had passed out.

Annie checked Billy's pulse—still alive. As Annie pondered what to do, she saw headlights coming down the road. Standing tall, she jumped up and down, waving her arms for the vehicle to stop, not realizing that any car driving by would see the flames lighting up the darkness.

As the truck stopped, Annie hurried to the passenger window and asked the man who looked like a farmer if he knew any first aid. "Yes, Ma'am."

Annie told the driver of the man's condition, ordered him to stay with the man, and ran to her car to go get help. She pulled into the drive of the first farmhouse she spotted, about a mile down the road, and asked to use the phone—there had been an accident. After making the 911 call and getting directional help from the elderly farmer and his wife as to the location of the accident, Annie thanked them, and drove back down the driveway to turn on to Pebble Creek Road.

In a moment of panic and fear, Annie Sinclair, being 18 and foolish, turned right towards home, rather than left to go back to the scene. She saw the ambulance and fire truck zoom by her, reached home without further incident, showered, and crawled into bed.

Each day thereafter she vowed to tell her parents and to go tell the police what had happened, but she never did. Surprisingly, there was virtually no newspaper or TV coverage about the crash, only that a UVa student had crashed on Pebble Creek Road. The driver suffered a broken leg and had been released from the hospital the next day with minor burns. The police were looking for a Good Samaritan. They knew there was another car involved but Billy insisted that he couldn't remember anything, which was mostly true, but he was also protecting his Angel. She obviously didn't want to be found. The first-aid farmer in the truck and the old couple at the farmhouse were no help in describing the "young girl" who had saved Billy Hamilton' s life. And they couldn't give the police a description of the car she was driving. Announcements in the newspaper looking for a Good Samaritan went unanswered.

For some time after the crash, when Annie the Angel ran errands in town or was just walking around Charlottesville, she would search through the crowds of people hoping to recognize and meet the man she had saved. But she didn't have a very clear image in her mind of the man's appearance. After awhile, life moved on and Annie kept the secret of that night buried deep inside for thirty years. Not even John was aware that his wife, on the night of her high school graduation, had saved a man's life.

Billy Hamilton made the most of his second chance. When he recovered from the crash, he transferred to the University of Richmond and sat out his junior year to concentrate on academics. He attacked his studies with newfound passion, and in his senior year played on one of the best basketball teams in Spiders' sports history, making it to the NCAA tournament. Billy Pelican returned to Charlottesville for medical school at UVa, but could never locate the young woman who had given him a second chance at living. Of course, it was very difficult to find a Good Samaritan, whose name he knew only as Annie the Angel.

Twenty-Three

ANNIE'S FINAL RUN

Annie woke for her last full day at White Horse Island. She didn't have the specifics planned out, only that she was going to make the most of it, capped off by the fun clambake that evening. She knew she had touched, felt, and played her way to that deep felt sense of herself that had been missing for a long time. She felt that she really knew what it was like to experience herself, not just going through the motions of life, not just knowing about. She planned to take this rediscovered feel of living into more physical activity, eating lighter, and re-establishing her relationship with her family, especially with John and Dylan. She also had ideas for members and her staff. She trusted that she could do it and that she would like doing it.

Annie put on her swimsuit and then her running attire over the top—a barefoot run along the beach and then body surfing, a great way to begin her final day. She felt revitalized as she stretched in the sand, another glorious day on White Horse Island. Annie began her final, shoeless run towards the pier as the sun began its daily skyward trek. Her mind floated. Why do I feel so different? Will it last? I wonder how Sam is doing? How can I play with John and Dylan? What happens if things fall apart when I get back? How could I recreate or bring this White Horse Island experience to my staff? To my members? She shifted through these questions, not really answering any of them, but playing around with possibilities.

As Annie neared the pier, she shifted her focus back to running, speeding up just a bit as the excitement of reaching the halfway point sparked both her mind and body. Near the end of the pier she spotted Doc sitting on a bench with Obi resting below.

"Hey, Doc. Hey, Obi," Annie said, drawing near. "Watchya doing?"

Doc, with his shades in the usual spot, turned slowly to face Annie, as it sometimes took him awhile to generate energy in the morning. Obi looked up, hoping that this might be someone that would play with him, tail wagging.

"Hi Annie. Just contemplating the day. Good to see you up and at 'em," said Doc.

"Can I sit with you?" asked Annie.

"Sure, if I can run back with you?"

"Sure. That would be great."

Annie petted Obi as she sat next to Doc and looked out to sea. What a peaceful place. She didn't want to leave.

"Hey Doc, can I ask a question about this process I've been experiencing?" Annie asked.

"I would be disappointed if you didn't," said Doc.

"This has been an experience of a lifetime," said Annie, "I truly mean that. I feel so fortunate that you guys chose me."

"Billy chose you," Doc said. "I'm just along for the whilds—W… H…I…L…D…S…White…Horse…Island…Life…Detective… Service—ride."

"Okay, Billy chose me…Hey, that's kind of cute with the detective thing…But, I guess, the entire experience seems kind of mystical, like a fantasy. What do I do when I get back to reality tomorrow and the next day? You know what I mean?"

"You mean when you get back to the real world?" asked Doc.

"I guess."

"I would be an expert if I answered that correctly, which I can't," said Doc. "What I will say is that the missing link can be found in what you brought with you to White Horse Island."

"What I brought with me?"

"C'mon, let's run back," Doc said, standing up and stretching. "You can play detective and mull it over on the run back."

"Doc, seriously, that's your answer?" Annie asked.

"Yep, let's go. C'mon, Obi."

The run back was relatively quiet, with Annie lost in her thoughts wondering about the things she had brought with her to White Horse Island.

"Man, I will miss these runs," Doc exclaimed as they reached the shoreline across from the shack.

"Awesome," said Annie, finishing a little behind Doc.

"So when are you leaving?" asked Doc.

"I need to leave tomorrow. My Y is sponsoring a charity run on Saturday and I want to be there."

"Yeah, I'm leaving tomorrow morning…early. I want to get back to watch my son's football game."

"Friday Night Lights," said Annie. "What position does your son play?"

"He's the quarterback. The team is young so they're taking their lumps. But I see some promise. Does your son play any sports?"

"Well, he likes basketball. But he hasn't really applied himself to it. Middle school was rough. I'm hoping high school will be better for him. He's a freshman."

"Maybe you can hook him up with Billy."

"Maybe."

Annie prepped for her body surfing experience but Doc's challenge was tugging at her.

"This is driving me crazy, Doc," Annie blurted out. "Something I brought with me can help me turn what I've been doing here into reality in Charlottesville?"

"Well, I don't know if it's *the* answer, but it is the link that connects everything together."

"What, my running shoes, my swimsuit, my phone, my laptop—"

"I guess all of those things could work. I was thinking more about something you can look at but hide away."

"Something I can look at but hide away? Well, my swimsuit falls into that category."

"Good one," Doc said, "but don't do that anymore. You're inviting judgment. I wasn't thinking of any of the things you mentioned. Think about it some more in between bodysurfs. I'm going in for some breakfast. If I don't see you, enjoy your last day. You are off to a great start."

"I'll see you tonight at the clambake," said Annie.

"Not if I see you first," Doc said, as he headed for the shack. Doc grabbed the ball from Obi's mouth and threw it towards the shack. Obi dashed through the sand to once again save his ball from being alone.

Annie walked into the water up to her hips and then dove in, still thinking about something that she brought with her that she could look at but hide away.

Twenty-Four

A PEARL OF PICTURES

While Annie bodysurfed, Doc showered and then ate more of Billy's homemade yogurt packed with fresh black raspberries. How does he get this fruit? Doc wondered. While Doc was eating, Billy came out of his hole and showed Doc what he had been working on.

"So you took all of her photos, scanned them, and then put together this watchyamacallit?" Doc asked.

"*Pearl of Pictures*," said Billy with a note of playful disdain at Doc's use of words.

Billy hit play on the iMovie for Doc and a picture of Annie as a young child showed up in the middle of the screen, and then photos capturing her life, appearing chronologically, began to appear one by one, ultimately forming multiple rings of photos growing around the centered picture. The pictures included ones with her parents and brother, her friends, Kate and Sam, playing tennis, and early pictures of her own family—John, Dylan, and Maggie.

"Annie will love this. So this ties into refueling the feel, right?" Doc asked.

"Yeah, but it's so much more than that," said Billy. "It's a way to remind Annie that these pictures capture her natural way of being, her promise being fulfilled. That if she keeps playing *The Game With No Name*, her spot will keep growing outward and her life will generate meaning and informed energy. I like the pearl because it's round. That's where my notion of the spot comes from. Natural pearls, not cultured pearls, grow this way and are quite rare. So when I'm talking about the spot, I'm mostly comparing it to the growth process of a natural pearl."

"That's interesting. I remember when you first introduced this idea to me, I went and looked for pictures of pearls," said Doc. "The natural ones have multiple rings of…what's that material called…?"

"Nacre," said Billy. "A cultured pearl has a very thin ring of nacreous coating. A natural pearl is one hundred percent nacre or pearl and each one varies in size and shape. Perfectly round is very rare. That's why Annie's picture movie is the *Pearl of Pictures*, rings of pureness, wonder, like a natural pearl.

"Or like a pelican flying," said Doc. "So we'd rather be around birds and natural pearls. I still wonder why it's so difficult for most of us to play *The Game With No Name*. I know I've asked this before, but if things like natural pearls and birds flying are so natural, why don't we do what should come natural to us?"

"Because our culture is not set up for each of us to naturally touch and feel that spot. We end up playing The Game set up by others, not our own *Game With No Name*. And The Game tells us we're not good enough, not strong enough, not pretty enough. It steals the stillness, fills the space, breaks the silence. No one can win The Game because it's a game of what we are not."

"That's what health and fitness does to us," said Doc, getting excited. "It's part of The Game. Exercise, eat right, do yoga, control your stress, get the recommended hours of sleep, and on and on and on."

"What's The Game?" Billy asked, pushing Doc.

Doc thought about it. "Not to die," he said. "We can't win that game."

"Right," Billy said. "And it's not much fun, so people don't play it very well."

"But if we begin to play *The Game With No Name*, if we play our game, we touch and feel our spot," Doc said. "We begin to reknow it, to trust it, and we naturally create and do things that fuel or refuel our spot, to keep it growing."

"Yes, but I think the real danger of The Game, as it pertains to health and fitness, is that people pursue these activities to help them win The Game, a game they can't win. They are told that if they would only listen to the experts, the consultants, the personal coaches they can win The Game. But they're playing the wrong game. They will mostly fail and not commit or engage because they know deep down, it's not their game."

Billy's statement reminded Doc of why college students don't engage. "Damn, it's so simple," said Doc. "I played The Game for so many years, rubbing his temples as if to exorcise all of his demons from The Game. But now that I can see it, now that I've felt more of my spot lately, it seems ridiculous how I have tried to be things I am not."

"I agree, I think you are beginning to play your own game," Billy said.

"Some people would say it's being selfish," said Doc, playing devil's advocate, "especially chairs and deans."

"Bullshit," said Billy, slamming his fist down on the kitchen table. "Don't listen to those people. They are playing The Game and want you to play it with them. They want you to worry, to be afraid. People who play their own game, *The Game With No Name*, are the ones who are going to save this country, the world. They are the ones who can create the informed energy to share with others less fortunate. They are the ones who will light up the darkness."

Doc was taken aback by Billy's tirade. Billy still had the fire. He was on a mission to change the world one person at a time, starting with Annie. And he was somehow going to do it using a shack as life detective headquarters on White Horse Island. Billy had once told Doc he was so relentless because The Game is even more so.

Billy took his *Pearl of Pictures* and headed back to his hole of a room. "By the way, I'll need you to pick up some stuff for the clambake tonight," Billy said, just before closing his door.

I guess this isn't a good time to discuss the issue of the weight scale at the Spa, Doc thought. Doc got out his pen and paper and wrote "*Clambake List.*" Obi looked up, just wanting someone to throw him the damn ball.

———&———

A nnie headed back to the big house with her chair, book, and towel in tow, still pondering Doc's quasi-riddle. The run and bodysurfing had been stellar. She would miss Doc and Billy. Only knowing them a few days, they felt like family. She was fearful of not being able to continue what she had started without them.

"Annie, Annie," a voice disrupted her thoughts.

"Annie, hey, Annie," the voice said again. This time Annie was aware that the voice was coming from behind her, and she turned to see Chrissie walking on the path at a fast clip, obviously taking a fitness walk.

"Hi Chrissie. Good walk?" Annie asked.

"Yes, thanks. I saw you and thought maybe we can play some tennis later."

"Great timing. This is my last day. I would love to play. What time?"

"Oh, I don't know. Early afternoon, two o'clock?"

"Perfect. Can you bring a racket for me?"

"Sure. Okay, I'll see you then," said Chrissie, who continued her speed walking on the path that would take her all the way to town.

Annie purposefully walked around to the front of the house. She remembered seeing a sign on the front of the shack and wanted to get a second look. Walking past the swing, she noticed the shingle hanging clumsily from a nail on the front door:

The White Horse Island Life Detective Service
Clues for the Clueless

Annie stopped and smiled. I guess I was pretty clueless when I arrived here, Annie thought. I didn't even see that sign the first night. She didn't feel that way now. She turned and headed to enter the big house via the front door.

Sam and Kate were sitting on the sofa with pictures scattered all over—on the coffee table, the floor, and the sofa.

"Sam, you're back. Thank goodness," Annie said. "How are you feeling?"

"I feel fine. Harry stayed with me at the hospital. He just dropped me off about thirty minutes ago. I'm ready for another day of excitement at White Horse Island."

"Let's hope not as exciting as—hey, these are all of my pictures," Annie said, finally recognizing the images. "What are you doing with all of them?"

"Well, Sam just wanted something to cheer her up and all I could come up with was your pictures," said Kate. "Doctor said no alcohol so a margarita was out. You don't mind do you?"

"No, no, I'm glad you are putting them to good use," as she sat down and picked up some of the photos. "Better then hiding them away in that box."

It took Annie a few seconds for the answer to Doc's riddle to register. But as she thumbed through the photos, it dawned on her that the pictures were what she had brought with her and had hid away.

"You guys just solved a riddle for me," said Annie.

"What do you mean?" asked Kate.

Annie informed her two friends of her fear about taking back what she had begun to touch and feel at White Horse Island and keeping it going in Charlottesville. She then told them about Doc's riddle and how her pictures were the answer to it.

"That just seems too easy," said Sam. "How can pictures do all of that?"

"I don't know, Sam, but there are some powerful images in here," said Kate. "Why hide those images? Why not put them to work for you?"

"You're starting to sound like Doc," said Annie.

"I've got an idea," said Kate. "I'll pretend I'm Doc doing one of his debriefs and we'll talk you through it, Annie."

"I don't know…" Annie answered, hesitant.

"Great idea, Kate," said Sam, as she reached in her purse and pulled out her sunglasses. "Here, put these on for full effect."

Kate put on the sunglasses and turned to Annie. She leaned forward and rubbed her hands, mimicking Doc.

Sam and Annie roared.

"So, Annie, do you have a few minutes to play a game with pictures?" Kate said, as she began the role play. "C'mon, we'll play *The Game With No Name* and then debrief."

Sam and Annie roared again. Kate sounded just like Doc.

"Okay, Doc, I'll do it," Annie said, playing along.

"Well…uh…in this game, we have all of these pictures from your life…and…uh…we pick one…and…uh…you have to explain how the picture connects to your spot."

"Ewwwwwww," said Sam, "I still think that word is perverted."

"Shut up, Sam, or I won't save your skinny ass next time," said Kate.

Sam and Annie roared.

"Sam, pick a picture for Annie," ordered the fake Doc. "Annie, keep your eyes closed. No peeking. I want you to be surprised."

"Why?" asked Annie.

"No questions. Can't you tell I'm making this up as I go," said the fake Doc.

Annie and Sam roared again. Kate had Doc nailed.

Sam looked around, picked a photo, and handed it to Doc, who handed it to Annie.

Annie felt the photo. She missed that feeling of holding a photograph. Digital had ended that experience.

"Now…uh…when I tell you to open your eyes, not yet, tell us your reaction to the image," said Doc.

Annie nodded.

"Okay…uh…open," said Doc.

Annie saw the three of them. They were standing next to Sam's "new" Honda civic, wearing cut off jean shorts and t-shirts, flexing their muscles for the camera. They must have been sixteen or seventeen with hair down to their butts and smiles out to their ears.

"Well, this makes me feel strong," said Annie.

"Good….good…tell us more. What else?" asked Doc.

"It reminds me that we had a bond that was so strong that it can never be broken. That we were wild and free, like wild horses, full of dreams about our lives.

"I like that," said Doc.

"Me too," said Sam, who was actually serious. "Keep going."

"And that I still have the promise to live those dreams. This picture reminds me that I can still feel strong and free no matter what the world throws at me and my friends, no matter what obstacles appear before me."

Sam and Kate clapped.

"So…uh…Annie…what do you think was the point of this game? How did playing it make you feel?" asked Doc.

"I feel re-energized. Focused. Like I'm not tired."

"Informed energy," said Kate, who was now serious as she recalled one of their chats with Doc.

"Yes, Kate, informed energy. Exactly. These pictures are ways to refuel the energy, to keep the spot growing."

"Speaking of spot," said Sam, "Let's find our spot on the beach. This is Annie's last day to enjoy the beach and we leave on Saturday."

"I'll make sandwiches," said Kate.

"I'll clean up the pictures," said Annie.

That took awhile. Afterwards, Annie vowed to herself never to hide the photos again and then went out to join Kate and Sam on the beach.

Twenty-Five

REFLECTION ON THE BEACH

The one thing the three women had planned on doing the most during their reunion vacation, they ended up doing the least—lying on the beach. But the best friends made the most of their last hurrah on the beach of White Horse Island—they built a sandcastle, Annie gave Sam a few bodysurfing lessons, and they watched the pelicans while munching on Kate's sandwiches.

Every now and then Annie would look over to the shack and see Billy and a few of his friends—she recognized Ian and Mac—preparing the firepit for the evening's clambake. The guys reminded Annie of a bunch of busy beavers only they were using shovels, stones, wood, and what looked like seaweed. She didn't see Doc anywhere.

As she watched, one of the things Annie realized was that while at White Horse Island she hadn't really thought much about food. When she was hungry she ate. And she didn't gulp down any coffee after that first day. And no snacks. When she was at home or at work, she would stop at Starbucks for her morning coffee and maybe order a muffin or coffee cake on top of her breakfast. In the afternoons she would have more coffee with a snack. Evenings were a crapshoot for dinner based on the hectic family schedule.

"Hey guys," Annie said, as she turned back to Kate and Sam, both of whom were lying on their backs, eyes closed, worshipping the sun.

"Can't you see we're sleeping," said Kate.

"Can't you see I'm still recovering from my day of terror," said Sam.

"Yea, yea, hey, I've got a question for you two," said Annie.

"Oh boy, here we go again," said Kate, as she grabbed Sam's arm to help her sit up. They both kept their legs straight and placed their hands in the sand behind them for support. "Did you see more White Horses or something?"

"What?" asked Sam.

"Never mind," said Kate. "I'll tell you later. I can tell Annie's ready for more self-exploration."

"Well, it's mostly just an observation," said Annie. "Do you realize that since I've been here I haven't had any snacks, only one cup of coffee, and ate fruit and yogurt almost every morning."?

"Well, let's review shall we," said Kate. "That's probably because you were having too much fun shooting arrows at fake animals, running on the beach, bodysurfing, getting high, getting whacked in the head by a Frisbee, playing a freaky game of tennis by moonlight, playing in a kiddie pool, hiking up dunes, and making a mad dash out of the Spa…did I leave anything out?"

Annie hadn't told Kate or Sam about the narrow escape from a pack of stampeding wild horses.

"Hello," said Sam. "You forgot hang gliding?"

"Oh, yes, and let's not forget the hang gliding experience where one of your two best friends in the whole wide world almost got killed. I think you've been a little too busy to snack."

"Very nice review, Kate," said Sam.

"Yes, very nice, Kate," said Annie. "But I'm always busy at home and work, and yet I find time for coffee, snacks, and I rarely eat fruit, and… and…I've slept better here than at home."

"Well, I've said it before," said Sam, "you are on vacation."

"I know. You could be right, Sam. But you said it Kate," said Annie. "I've been having too much fun. I've been playing and I haven't needed that other stuff."

"Could be," said Kate. "Why not?"

"Doc and I had a discussion where he talked about there comes a time, like a transcendent moment, where you reconnect so deeply into who you are that you begin to connect experiences like exercise and eating foods that make you feel light, that you'll naturally be attracted to those behaviors that feed this source of energy. You'll change behavior without really trying to change behavior."

"Isn't that kind of like one of the Pelican's Principles: Start with what's right about you?" said Kate.

"Pelican's Principles?" asked Sam.

"We'll tell you later," replied Kate and Annie in unison.

"Well, do you think you've had a transcendent moment?" asked Kate.

"You know what I think," said Annie. "I think this whole week has been my transcendent moment. For whatever reason, I was drawn to White Horse Island to lose weight. It was my moment. I want to thank you guys for staying with me on this. I know it hasn't been easy."

"Well, someone's got to be there for a crazy woman," said Sam. "Speaking of crazy, I think I'm in love with Harry, and it's not just because the sex has been great."

"SAM," said Kate and Annie.

"But seriously, I'm coming back for Thanksgiving," Sam added.

"Sam, that's great. Harry seems like a great guy," said Kate.

"Yes, Sam, you make a great couple," said Annie. Annie had noticed a difference in Sam. She wondered what Billy would think. He probably already knew.

"Oh my gosh, the time," said Annie, looking at the time on her phone. "I promised Chrissie I would play tennis with her at two. Would you guys mind? I've been wanting to play real tennis on those clay courts and—"

"No problem," interrupted Kate. "Save your breath. Sam and I can drive into town for one more round of shopping."

Sam nodded.

"Okay, great," said Annie, as she gathered up her beach gear. "Just remember the clambake tonight. I want you guys to come."

"Wouldn't miss it," said Sam. "I'd love to hang out with that little pecker and chest man."

"SAM," Annie shouted as she hurried to the house to change.

Twenty-Six

Tennis, Anyone?

Annie jogged over to the tennis courts, a towel draped over her shoulders. She was excited to get back on the courts and play some real tennis, although she definitely had fun playing *Turn Tennis* the other night. Her body felt energized and she wondered how she had let tennis out of her life for the past 20 years or so. She tried to get the kids interested but Maggie didn't have the eye-hand coordination; Dylan turned into Godzilla on the courts and made playing stressful; and John wouldn't give up the competition, even against his own wife. He acted like an asshole and never eased up. He was just one of those unlikable tennis players. In the end, Annie just let it go and her body followed suit.

Annie spotted Chrissie on one of the far courts and waved.

"Hi Annie," said Chrissie. "Glad you could make it."

"Thanks for inviting me. I've never played on clay courts."

"You'll love it and so will your knees," Chrissie said, handing Annie one of her rackets. "How do you want to do this?"

"Well, maybe just hit around for awhile and then play a set. That will probably be all my body can handle."

"Sounds good to me," said Chrissie.

Chrissie was a great playing partner. She hustled after errant balls and stroked shots that made Annie move just enough to hit both forehands and backhands, but didn't exhaust her. Annie could tell her own movements were slower and she began to breathe heavier after about forty-five minutes. Chrissie still seemed fresh. Her movements were lithe and nimble, and she expended little needless energy.

"Why don't you try some serves," said Chrissie, give you a little rest.

"Great idea," said Annie. Surprisingly, she felt strong serving. Chrissie kept saying, "nice" or "looks good." Chrissie's serves were slower than Annie's but had lots of spin. And her placement was impeccable into either the Ad or Deuce court. Annie thought Chrissie was serving much better today than the other night, of course, serving under moonlight with an old Kramer racket weren't ideal conditions.

"Let's take a break," Chrissie said, after about an hour. "I brought some water in a cooler."

Chrissie got out a couple of paper cups from her bag and handed one to Annie. The water was beautifully cold and Annie relished the sips and the rest. They both sat on the side bench and toweled off.

"You've got game," said Chrissie. "Do you play in a league or anything?"

"No, I played in high school and we had a great team. I played a little in college and early in my marriage but then stopped."

"Why?"

"Good question. I guess life just took over," Annie said.

"What do you mean?"

"You know, work, kids. I just didn't make the time and kind of forgot about it after awhile."

"Is that the real reason?"

"I think so."

"You're sure? My story is similar but I don't think I stopped because of work and kids. I stopped because I didn't do enough to find the right people to play with."

"What do you mean?" Annie asked.

"Well, my kids disliked tennis and so did my husband. I just didn't have any friends to play with so I gave up."

"Hey, me too. I think that's right. No friends. No 'tennis, anyone?'"

"When my husband died a few years ago, I retired, and moved here permanently. After we had vacationed here so many summers, I just fell in love with the place. My kids are all grown and I love the beach. I figured why not."

"I'm…I'm so sorry about your husband," said Annie.

"It's okay. He had colon cancer but we had a great life together before that. I just hold on to the good memories."

"If you don't mind me asking, how old are you?"

"Sixty two."

Annie just about fell off the bench. "I thought you were my age," said Annie. "I'm forty eight. You look incredible. Wow…Oh…I'm sorry…you were going to tell me how you got back into tennis."

"It's simple, really. When I moved here, my first summer, I saw a poster for a women's tennis league looking for players. I decided that I had missed tennis long enough. I signed up. Guess who my team's coach was?"

"I have no idea?"

"Billy."

"Billy Pelican? I mean, Billy Hamilton is your coach?"

"He's been helping us for a few years now. He would help us in the summers the first couple of years and when he moved down here permanently my game really took off. I've improved so much. It's incredible. We made it to nationals a few years ago…and won. But the friendships I have formed with my teammates and the women we meet when we travel to tournaments can't be matched by any title."

"That sounds like so much fun."

"It is. The competition is based on your level of ability and age so the matches are almost always competitive and fair. You have to play your best to win. I think you would really enjoy the experience."

"I know I would. I've heard of these leagues but I never really pursued them."

"You should check it out when you get back. I guarantee that you will make friends for life."

"I will. Thank you so much for sharing your story."

"No problem. Now, are you ready to get whopped?"

Annie tried her best, but she was rusty. Her serve kept her in the set but Chrissie was quicker and more fit, and won going away, 6-2. After the handshake, Chrissie offered Annie some more water, which she gladly accepted. She was dripping with sweat.

"Again, you've got a really nice game," said Chrissie. "You've got power. That's not something you can teach."

"Thank you," said Annie. "If you don't mind me asking, what has Billy helped you with the most?"

"Not too much technically," replied Chrissie. "I would say trusting myself, trusting my game. Not being afraid to go for it when the game is on the line.

"Yea, that seems to be what others say as well," said Annie.

"I guess, he just helps me be me," said Chrissie. "He gets right on the court with me and asks, 'How did that feel, How does this feel?' Just lots of questions that force me to pay attention and make observations. It's kinda simple really."

"Well, I'd better be going," said Annie. "Are you coming to the clam-bake tonight at Billy's?"

"Sure, wouldn't miss it."

They walked off the courts together and then Chrissie headed to her car in the lot, while Annie headed toward the path by the Spa. She spotted a Jeep pulling into the Spa's entrance circle. It was Harry's Jeep, but Billy was driving.

"Tennis, anyone?" Billy said to greet her.

Annie came over. "Hello, Doctor Pelican, what are you doing with Harry's Jeep?"

"Actually, it's my Jeep. I let Harry borrow it. I usually just ride my bike. Harry went into town with Kate and Sam and I've got a few hours to kill."

"What about the clambake?" Annie asked.

"Ian and Mac and Doc are on it. Want to go for a drive?" Billy thought of that night thirty years when a fateful drive brought them together.

"I'm all sweaty," said Annie.

"Ah, that's okay. Breeze will dry you off. C'mon, I don't bite."

"Where we goin'?" asked Annie, as she climbed in and closed the door.

"North," Billy said and peeled out.

Twenty-Seven

DRIVING ON THE BEACH

"How was the tennis?" asked Billy as he headed towards Corolla on Highway 12.

"I'd say it was the most fun I've had since I've been here but then everything I've done has been fun."

"Even getting hit in the head by a Frisbee?"

"Well, that was fun just *before* I got hit by DJ. Where are we going again?"

"Where I grew up," said Billy. "Takes about a half hour. I would just relax and enjoy the ride."

Billy gave good advice as Annie felt the wind whip her air and she breathed in the salt air. She caught glimpses of the sound to her left.

As they neared Corolla, Billy pointed to the left. "That's where I spent a lot of my youth, the Whalehead Club. We'll stop in on our way back. I know the caretaker, Gus. He'll let us roam around a bit after hours. I just want to show you one more thing before you head back tomorrow."

Annie nodded. She was just taking it all in. The land around the Whalehead Club looked pristine from the glimpse she had as Billy zoomed by.

A few miles further and Annie began to see trees lining a forest to her left and then the ocean was visible through snippets of views in between the oceanfront homes on her right. Billy made a gradual turn to the right and the world opened up—it looked like they would drive straight into the ocean. Surrounded by trees and shrubs and sand and water. Emptiness, nothingness, silence. Annie felt like she was at the gates of heaven. Billy stopped the car. "I need to let some air out of the tires. You can get out and stretch a minute if you want."

Annie got out and walked toward the ocean. A few people were milling about. Some of them were walking along the beach. She noticed the fence.

"Okay," Billy said. "We're ready."

Annie headed back and hopped in the Jeep. "Where are we headed?"

"We're going to take a drive on the beach," Billy said. "See if we can find us some wild horses."

Annie shook a bit, thinking of the close call she had the other night.

"Is that why the fence is there, to keep the horses in?" Annie asked.

"Yea, they just had to protect the horses from themselves and stupid people," Billy said. "It goes from the ocean all the way to the sound on the other side."

"So how were the horses down by us the other night?" Annie asked.

"I have no idea," said Billy. "Maybe you attract danger."

Annie gave Billy another friendly swat across his arm. Life detective, Annie wondered, you create more mysteries than you solve, Billy Pelican. Wild horses, White Horses. Annie was trying to determine if it was all real or just some fantasy she had created in her mind. Doubt was creeping in.

"This is beautiful," said Annie as Billy headed over closer to the water to drive on the hard-packed sand.

"I agree. I hope it doesn't go away at some point. The number of homes in here just keeps growing. If paved roads ever go in, the horses are finished."

A few vehicles passed them heading to Corolla and everyone waved.

"So how do you feel about going back?" Billy asked.

"Usually near the end of a vacation, I'm ready to get back to the real world."

"But not this time?"

"Yes and no. Yes, because I'm excited about continuing some things based on what I experienced here for myself, my family, and with my job, and, No, because I feel like I've just tapped the surface of what White Horse Island could help me create for myself and the people around me."

"Well, you can always come back for a refresher," said Billy. "White Horses are always willing."

Again, Annie had that feeling of something not quite right, a feeling that all of it was a mirage.

"Okay, let's talk about this right now," Annie said. "Stop the car. This is driving me a little nuts."

Annie got out of the car, took off her tennis shoes, and walked towards the ocean, towards heaven. Billy followed.

"How come I don't see them?" asked Annie.

"Don't see what?" asked Billy.

"The White Horses. How come I see them sometimes and not others? Kate and I saw them the other day walking to the Spa, which by the way opens up a whole other can of worms about the damn scale in there. Don't even get me started on that. The fact that Kate and I have both seen the White Horses makes me think we're both a little nuts. I mean there can't really be White Horses coming out of the ocean. I mean I'd like to believe, but c'mon."

Annie turned around to see Billy's reaction.

"Kate saw them?" said Billy. "That's great."

Annie threw up her arms in exasperation. "Who are you Billy Pelican? What are the White Horses?"

"I've always been able to see the White Horses," Billy said, "ever since my grandfather showed me how to find them years ago. I've learned not to question it. My grandfather told me that White Horse Island is a magical place. I've always believed that. I've just decided it's time to share what they can do for other people besides me."

"But why me? Why now?" asked Annie. "What did I do to deserve the White Horses?"

Billy didn't want to tell the whole story, not now.

"Let's just say you are special beyond your wildest imagination," Billy said. "And that's why the White Horses appeared to you. You were ready to play, to commit to the process of being weightless. You just have to trust me, that's the truth."

Annie took a deep breath.

"And you've done it, Annie, you've done it," Billy continued. "Weight loss is about consuming less—restrictions, cutting back, working harder. Weightless is about creating the life you like. You're ready to create that life right now, the life that *you* like."

"But I'm scared. What if I can't do it? What if this has all been some kind of wild fantasy and I wake up and it never happened? What if I wake up in Charlottesville and forget everything. What if I just go on living the way I've been living? I can't take that life anymore. I hate it."

"That won't happen," said Billy.

"But how can you be so sure?"

"Because this is what I do for a living and I'm good at it. I know. I don't know why the White Horses come when I call. They just do. My grandfather told me never to question the magic. I'm telling you, you've seen them because you're ready."

Annie looked up at Billy, hesitating. "You're still an asshole, Billy Pelican."

Billy laughed.

"So all of this has been real? You're not shitting me or anything?"

"It's all been real. You made it happen. Things happen in life that you can't always explain with scientific research or logical thinking. For example, why are these horses walking toward us at this very moment?" Billy asked.

Annie turned and saw a pack of wild horses meandering their way. She jumped and hid behind Billy.

Billy laughed again. "They're harmless. They're just enjoying the cool breeze and no bugs bothering them."

They watched as the horses strolled by a few feet away.

"They're beautiful," Annie whispered, "but I like the White Horses better."

They kept their eyes on the horses until they were a good stone's throw away. "Here, hop on," said Billy, as he turned his hands out behind him.

Annie jumped on Billy's back and he carried her to the Jeep.

"Here we are your highness," said Billy, as he reached the car.

"Thank you, your majesty," said Annie, as she picked up her shoes and got back in the Jeep. Billy drove a few more miles up the coast, turned around after no further horse sightings, and headed back towards Corolla and the Whalehead Club, a short drive, interrupted by a quick stop to refill the Jeep's tires with air.

Twenty-Eight

The Whalehead Club

A little after six o'clock, Billy turned right near the Currituck Heritage Park sign, drove a short distance on Club Road, and parked in front of the Whalehead Club estate, which was now a museum. Annie, mesmerized by the beauty of the place, sat in awe. The entire property seemed like a shrine to peace and innocence.

"This is where my father lived for awhile with my grandfather after my grandmother passed away," Billy said.

"This…this was your grandfather's estate…all of this?" Annie asked.

"Yep, that was long before I came along," Billy said. "I lived for a short time in what is now the caretaker's residence." Billy pointed to the smaller house directly behind them. "I was too young to remember living there. We moved off the property when I was little."

"Why?

"Well, it's a long story but mostly because my grandfather got a little greedy and sold out to the government, and my father got stubborn. He never forgave my grandfather. I know that's why we moved to DC."

"I'm sorry to hear that. This place is majestic," said Annie.

"Before my grandfather died, he willed the entire property to Currituck County and they developed it into a place that people could visit. It's got everything: museum, wildlife education, you name it. Lots of people get married here."

"I can see why," said Annie. "The setting is breathtaking."

"I used to roam around here all day long when I was younger. There was a time when the place was abandoned. I had the run of the place. I would just explore. Come on, let's take a walk."

Billy and Annie walked some of the vast property and Billy even showed her the old schoolhouse—now a museum that paid homage to the wild horses—where his dad went to school for a few years, and the adjacent lighthouse. As they walked back, they crossed the historic Whalehead Bridge. Billy stopped at the peak. The setting sun had turned the sky into a glorious orange hue. It was, without a doubt, the prettiest sunset Annie had ever seen. It filled her with a renewed sense of hope and wonder about her life that she had not felt in a long time. She was ready to go back, to create that life. Now Annie was getting her second chance. This past week, Billy had returned the favor.

"C'mon," Billy said. "I want to show you one more thing." They walked over to the caretaker house, which had what looked like a large, detached garage next to it. Billy headed toward it. "This place is off limits to anyone but me," he said, as he pulled a key out of his pocket to unlock the padlock on the door.

Billy opened the door and held it so Annie could scoot in ahead of him.

"It's…it's a basketball hoop," Annie said, in disbelief. The area was just large enough to accommodate a high arcing jump shot and long enough to attempt three-pointers. The floor was all wood.

"This is where I learned to play," said Billy, who grabbed the basketball laying in the corner and starting dribbling. "This is my bliss station. I come here a few days a week to shoot. I guess it's my form of meditation."

"It's wonderful," said Annie, who imagined Dylan loving something like this, his own private sanctuary embedded within a much larger sanctuary. "But how did it get here?"

"Well, the original owner, my great grandfather, loved basketball, which was big up North when he had the Whalehead Club built. I guess this was his way of bringing the game with him. When I was younger, the original rim was still here. I've modernized it since I've come back for good." Billy shot and swished one.

"But how is it that you're still able to play here?" Annie asked.

"In his will, my grandfather explicitly stated that the shack and the basketball garage were to remain my property after the estate and the land was turned over to Currituck County. I think it was my grandfather's way of not letting go of the past, of redeeming himself for selling all of his other properties."

"Here, shoot a couple," Billy said, as he passed the ball to Annie. Annie took aim and misfired a few times until she moved closer and banked in a layup off of the new backboard.

"Here, you shoot," said Annie, as she passed the ball back to Billy. "I'm a tennis player."

Annie watched as Billy moved back and drained jumper after jumper. She rebounded for him and passed it back out after each swish. Billy's shot was pure, majestic. It looked effortless to Annie, like the ball was destined to go through the hoop each time.

"Beautiful," said Annie. "Doc says you didn't play much at UVa. That's hard to believe looking at that shot."

"Young and stupid," Billy said. "I lost my scholarship and then had to transfer. It all worked out in the end though. We'd better get going," as the Pelican drained one more jumper, "we've got a clambake to attend." Billy rolled the ball into a corner to rest until next time.

As they drove out of the park to head back for Annie's last hurrah at White Horse Island, the sky faded to a darker orange. Billy smiled. It was the very same color as his beloved basketball.

Twenty-Nine

THE CLAMBAKE

As Billy turned into the narrow, sandy drive of the shack, he didn't like what he saw: a Dare County Sheriff's car.

"Damn," he said, as pulled up alongside.

"What's wrong?" Annie asked. "Is it the firepit?"

"Probably," Billy said. "I just hope it's not Jimmy."

"Who's Jimmy?"

"Let's just say, I'm not on his good side."

"What's that awful sound?" asked Annie.

They walked around back and could hear Jackson Browne's *Pretender* coming out over the speakers, but that wasn't the awful sound. There was a group hovered around the fire pit.

As Billy and Annie approached the pit, they could see Jimmy and Sam in the middle of the group, arm in arm, belting out the song's lyrics. The group clapped as Jimmy stopped from exhaustion somewhere in the middle while Sam and Jackson continued together to the end of the song. Sam gave Jimmy a little hug and a peck on the cheek, spotted Annie, and waved with her left hand. Her right hand had a mug of beer in it. Sam left Jimmy, who headed back to his cruiser, and gave Annie a hug.

"Are you drunk?" asked Annie.

"A little," said Sam.

"Where's Kate?"

"Oh, I think she's shooting arrows with Ian and Mac. They're great guys."

"Shooting arrows?" Annie exclaimed. "O, Lord."

"Did you know you can't have firepits on the beach in White Horse Island?" asked Sam.

"Yes, I did know that," said Annie, who thought about Billy's question pertaining to breaking the rules. She had certainly broken a few this past week.

"Well, I took care of it," said Sam.

"What do you mean?" Annie asked.

"Jimmy was pissed when he arrived, mumbling something about Billy taking advantage of him and swearing that he was going to shut down the party and write him up. So…I just used all of my feminine whiles, introduced myself as the damsel in distress from yesterday, told him that Doc saved me, and that Billy was having a party in my honor. I asked Jimmy how he could in good conscience shut down such a great party. I made sure I talked using my pouty lips while my breasts *accidently* rubbed his badge. Then the *Pretender* came on and we just started singing. I love that song."

"I guess it worked," said Annie. "Thanks, Sam."

"Well, we couldn't have your last night at White Horse end on a sour note now could we?"

"I love you, Sam Suntan."

"I love you, Lil Orphan Annie."

They embraced one more time.

"Don't get too drunk," said Annie. "You're not supposed to be drinking."

"Last one, promise," said Sam, who spotted Harry and dashed over into his waiting arms.

Annie smiled, and saw Doc walking towards her with a plate in his hand.

"Here ya go," offered Doc, handing her the plate, "official White Horse Island clambake food."

"Thanks, Doc. I just realized I am famished."

"C'mon we'll go eat on the deck," said Doc, who went inside to turn down Jackson Browne, which elicited a groan from the crowd.

"This looks and smells amazing," said Annie, as she and Doc settled in the rickety, old chairs. "What is all this?"

"Well, as near as I can tell, there's lobster, clams, corn on the cob, red potatoes, smoked kielbasa sausage, in honor of my ancestors, and a few other things I'm not really sure of." Doc placed a container of garlic butter sauce on the table. "Dig in. Do you want a beer?"

"Sure."

Doc went and grabbed one from the cooler sitting on the deck. When he returned Annie was already attacking the lobster.

Annie's last supper was incredible. Doc shut up and let her eat, and they both finished around the same time.

"That was great," said Annie. "It seems like I ate a lot, but I don't feel stuffed. I love that feeling."

"Me too. So how was your ride with Billy?" Doc asked.

"Awesome," said Annie. "We saw some wild horses, and he showed me where he grew up. Did you know he has a basketball hoop in an old garage?"

"Wow, you must be special because he hasn't said or shown me any-thing like that," Doc said. "Speaking of special let's go inside for a minute. I want to show you something."

"Okay," said Annie.

Inside the shack, Doc had Annie sit at the kitchen table with Billy's laptop directly in front of her, powered up and ready to go. "Just watch," said Doc, as hit play.

The first picture of Annie as a small child playing in her backyard appeared on the screen, followed by the rings of pictures Billy had selected from her hidden stash. Annie watched in silence as her life unfolded, full of smiles and friends and dreams of youth. It ended with the final ring including pictures from the family she had started with John almost twenty years ago.

Billy handed Annie a tissue. "Play it again," she ordered, as she dabbed her eyes.

The *Pearl of Pictures* silent movie played again in its entirety, followed by moments of silence.

"It's my spot isn't it," declared Annie.

"Yes," Doc replied.

"And it's growing, isn't it," she said.

"Yes. That's why you brought the pictures, isn't it," Doc said. "Because you believed that the promise was still there, buried deep inside."

Annie nodded. "Did Billy make this?"

"Of course, do you think I have the skill to pull this off?" Doc asked, already knowing the answer.

Annie laughed. She didn't even bother to ask how Billy got the pictures.

"Can I have this somehow?" she asked.

"We already sent it to you. It's on your laptop. Now you can't hide these pictures anymore. Revisit them when you need to refuel. You can do a bunch of other things too, I mean, to revisit or refuel your feel, but we don't need to go over all of that now. This is a good start."

Annie stood up and gave Doc a strong embrace. "Thank you so much, Doc. I owe you my life."

"Don't make me cry," said Doc, "I don't have any tears. C'mon let's go out so you can say goodbye to all of your new friends."

Walking out to the beach, Annie spotted Kate, who was talking with Ian and Mac.

"Annie!" Kate exclaimed. "What a great way to end our vacation, uh."

"Hi Annie," said Ian and Mac.

"Hi guys, how was Kate at shooting? Did she hit any butts?"

"She almost hit mine," said Ian, who rubbed his ass for effect.

Everyone laughed as Doc plucked an arrow from Ian's quiver.

"Well, we'd better get going," said Mac. "It was a pleasure working on your case, Annie."

"The pleasure was all mine," said Annie, as she shook their hands before they drifted over towards the firepit.

"So one last lesson, ladies," said Doc, as he waved an arrow like a magical wand. "Watch closely."

"Okay, Doc, one last lesson," said Kate. "We've put up with you this long, what's a few more minutes."

"I thought you weren't an expert," said Annie.

"Well, just this one time," said Doc. "Just call me Doctor K."

Doc drew a circle in the sand with the arrow.

"So this is the circle of your life, Annie, your spot." At the top he wrote *Dream*, on the right at three o'clock he wrote *Prepare*, on the bottom of the circle he wrote *Obstacles*, and on the left at nine o'clock he wrote *Refuel*.

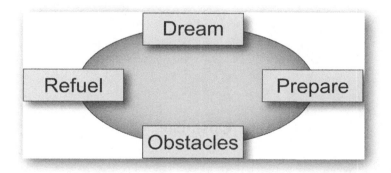

"That's the process for being weightless. How do you *like* to live? That's the Dream. How do you live it? That's Prepare. What might prevent or inhibit you from experiencing how you like to feel? That's Obstacles.

"You mean like judgment," Annie said.

"Yes," said Doc, "and how can you get that magic or feel back in your day quickly? That's Refuel."

"The *Pearl of Pictures*," Annie said.

Doc nodded.

"Uh?" said Kate.

"I'll tell ya later," said Annie.

Doc handed the arrow to Annie. "Now you draw the words that embody the process," he said, "the process that you experienced here at White Horse Island."

Without any conscious thought, Annie began to draw the words *inside* the circle, inside her spot: *Touch, Feel, Play, Know, Trust, Create.*

"How did she know to write those words?" asked Kate, amazed by how quickly Annie wrote them out. "What do they mean?"

"I got this, Doc," Annie said.

Doc nodded his approval.

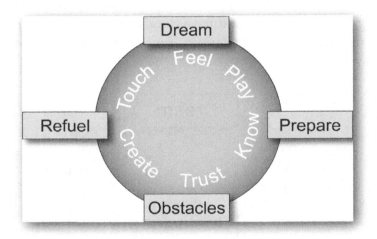

"Basically, my vacation started with *Touch*," Annie continued. "I was watching things that touched my spot, woke it up. Then I started to engage in activities, to begin to *Feel* my life at a deeper level. The White Horses reminded me that *Play* is the best way to touch, to feel my spot. So I played. Boy, did I play. This helped me begin to *Know* things for myself so that I can *Trust* my own process, and once all of that is in place, so to speak, I can begin to *Create* the life that I like, not want; to be weightless, rather than trying to lose weight."

Stunned silence.

"How'd I do, Doc?" Annie asked.

"Couldn't have said it any better myself," said Doc.

Kate started clapping. And then the clapping grew louder as others formed a circle around Annie. The clapping turned into an ovation.

Annie Sinclair Jackson was getting a standing ovation for the first time in her life.

Annie looked around at the faces in the circle. Everyone was there: DJ, the Frisbee guy, Chrissie, Harry, Ian and Mac, Sam and Kate, Doc and Billy, Lisa, the masseuse at the Spa, Dutch, the hang glider, the woman from the *White Horse Fish Company*, even Dolores, the receptionist from the YMCA and the FedEx guy were there clapping. Everyone who had touched her spot in some way over the past few days had formed a circle of life, and Annie was the spot inside.

The ovation climaxed and then subsided. The circle began to break up. Annie watched as Billy motioned for the White Horses to join him down by the water until only Kate, Doc, Sam, Harry, and Annie remained in the sand near the shack. It was time for the White Horses to return to the water, to play and dance together.

Billy shook each of their hands as they walked by him, ending with a special hug for Chrissie. They were all at the water's edge now. They all turned back one more time and waved to Annie.

Annie waved back, wanting to go with them but knowing she still had a life to create that she liked.

As they walked into the water, their bodies slowly transformed back into the White Horses, the magical White Horses that time and legend had forgotten. But Billy hadn't forgotten. He had called them and they had come, to serve their purpose, to live their Dream.

Annie watched as the White Horses played a bit longer and then vanished into the depths of the sea, waiting for the next time Billy called.

DEPARTURE

Billy watched from the front porch of the shack as Annie loaded her suitcase in the car. He saw her hug Kate and Sam, who came out to say their goodbyes. He watched as they talked for a few more minutes, probably about their next get together. Kate handed Annie the DVD she had forgotten to pick up from the coffee table.

Annie was happy that she had both the DVD and her *Pearl of Pictures* as mementos of her time at White Horse Island. Billy decided not to tell Annie that it was Bob who had taken all of the pictures and had put together her personalized DVD—some secrets are fun to keep. But there was one secret he wasn't going to keep from her any longer.

As Billy saw Kate and Sam head back inside, he grabbed the boxed present and walked towards Annie, who had turned in the direction of the shack for one last look.

They both smiled.

"Well, back to Charlottesville," said Annie, as Billy neared.

"At least it's a lot shorter drive than Doc's," said Billy. "His will take all day."

"I've got Doc's email. I'll stay in touch with him about some stuff we can work on with my Y," Annie said, and she meant it.

"That's a good idea," said Billy. "But don't forget about yourself in the process."

Billy pulled out the gift box he was holding behind his back and handed it to Annie. The box was wrapped in birthday-type paper, complete with a ribbon and bow that he and Doc had worked on last night.

"This is for you," Billy said.

Annie stared at the box, a very unexpected gift.

"It's beautiful. You shouldn't have," said Annie. "You've done so much for me."

"Well, aren't you going to open it?" Billy asked.

Annie hurriedly ripped through the wrappings and handed them to Billy. Opening the box she was shocked at what she saw. For a moment she was speechless.

"My quilt...the one that Granny Sinclair made for me. But how did you—".

Annie looked up at Billy.

Billy nodded.

Annie gasped, dropping the box with her quilt inside. She covered her mouth with her hands as she realized the thirty-year mystery was over. She had found her rescued man, or, rather, he had found her. Annie felt weak in the knees. She looked up at Billy's face again and began to sob uncontrollably. She wrapped her arms around him tight; she never wanted to let go of this big, beautiful man.

"I've been wondering about you for thirty years," Annie sobbed. "I stopped searching after a while because I didn't know how to find you."

"Well, you found me," said Billy, smiling, as he unhinged himself from Annie's grasp.

"I've always wondered what happened to you," said Annie. "I can't believe this is really happening. But...how...did...you...I mean...the quilt..."

"A couple of years ago, when I finally moved back to White Horse Island for good, I was sorting through some things in the closet of my bedroom."

"In the shack?" Annie asked.

"Yes, I stumbled upon the quilt that I had saved for all these years as a memory from that night when a young woman saved my life, when she gave me a second chance. I must have brought it with me on one of my visits from DC and just stuffed it in the closet.

"But I still don't understand. How did you find me from the quilt?" Annie asked.

"Well, when I unfolded the quilt this last time, for whatever reason, I noticed some embroidery in one of the corners. It was small and the color blended in with the quilt. It wasn't surprising that I had missed it before. Do you remember what your grandmother inscribed?"

"Oh…uh…'stay warm on cold nights' or something like that," Annie answered.

"Right," Billy said, as he picked up the quilt to show Annie the inscription:

Annie—stay warm on cold nights
Love, Grandma Sinclair
12-13-79

"Yes, I remember. It was a Christmas present from Granny," Annie said. "Boy, the inscription is hard to see."

"Yep, good ole 1979," Billy added. "Seems like yesterday."

Billy rubbed his hand over the embroidery. He loved the raised feel of those small stitches. He handed the quilt back to Annie. "Once I knew Annie the Angel's maiden name might be Sinclair," Billy said, "it was pretty easy via Classmates dot com and Facebook to find you—Annie Sinclair, now Annie Jackson, Charlottesville High School, 1981."

"So did you know that I was coming to White Horse Island this week?" Annie asked.

"Yes. I set it all up." Billy said.

"But how, how did you set it up?" Annie asked.

"Bob and I were talking one day and he told me about a phone conversation he had with a YMCA colleague in Charlottesville, Annie Jackson, who seemed very stressed and was looking for a vacation house on the Banks. Since I knew Annie Sinclair had married and was executive director of the Charlottesville Y, I knew he had been talking to my Annie. I told him to tell you that you could rent my house at a steep discount—".

"Wait a second," Annie interrupted, "first of all, Bob told me that he didn't know you or Doc, and second of all, are you kidding me, the house we rented this week is yours?"

"To confess, we had Bob lie to you about knowing me?"

"But why?" Annie asked.

"To create a little excitement, a little danger. It was our way of getting your attention. And, yes, the house you are renting is mine."

Annie was flabbergasted. "I...I...I don't know what to say. Why do you live in the shack and not this big, beautiful house?" asked Annie.

"I like the shack," Billy said. "It reminds me of my grandfather and the great times we had there. My grandfather owned all of this property and willed it to me. I had the big house built for special guests. You're the first official client of the *White Horse Island Life Detective Service* who is staying in the big house."

"Why didn't you tell me right away, like that first night when I met you and Doc?"

"This way was more fun," said Billy, flashing a mischievous grin.

"I...I don't know what to say," said Annie.

"You don't have to say anything. This was my way of paying you back some of what I owe. I tore up the check you made out to Bob and sent to him for the deposit. You don't owe me anything."

"I feel like I owe you everything. I feel like I've been living with this hole in my heart for the past thirty years," Annie said.

"Not anymore, you're growing your spot. You're fulfilling your promise," Billy said.

Annie wrapped the quilt around Billy and gave him another hug.

They talked for a few more minutes, as Annie wanted to know what happened to Billy and his life after the crash.

"You'd better get going," said Billy, finally, "you've got a great life to go live. Remember, you'll always have the White Horses when you need them."

Tears of joy and gratitude poured from Annie's heart. She gave Billy one more quick hug and then got in the car, placing the quilt softly on the passenger seat. She waved to Billy, tears flowing freely, and headed for home. As Annie drove over the Wright Memorial Bridge, she felt lighter, freer, like she was flying. Taking in the panoramic view, she spotted a pod of pelicans in the distance, and for no particular reason, flashed a smile as big and as wondrous as the Currituck Sound.

For the first time since high school, Annie Sinclair Jackson felt weightless.

About The Detectives (Aka Authors)

JAY KIMIECIK is a professor at Miami University (Oxford, OH) and slowly learning how to be his own life detective. He can be reached at kimiecjc@miamioh.edu.

DOUG NEWBURG travels around the United States and Canada working with athletes and business executives. He can be reached at dougnewburg@me.com.

Made in the USA
Coppell, TX
24 March 2025

47438231R00144